T0277638

Perimenopause

by Dr. Rebecca Levy-Gantt

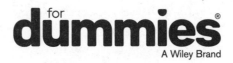
A Wiley Brand

Perimenopause For Dummies®

Published by: **John Wiley & Sons, Inc.,** 111 River Street, Hoboken, NJ 07030-5774, www.wiley.com

Copyright ©2024 by John Wiley & Sons, Inc., Hoboken, New Jersey

Published simultaneously in Canada

For general information on our other products and services, please contact our Customer Care Department within the U.S. at 877-762-2974, outside the U.S. at 317-572-3993, or fax 317-572-4002. For technical support, please visit https://hub.wiley.com/community/support/dummies.

Wiley publishes in a variety of print and electronic formats and by print-on-demand. Some material included with standard print versions of this book may not be included in e-books or in print-on-demand. If this book refers to media such as a CD or DVD that is not included in the version you purchased, you may download this material at http://booksupport.wiley.com. For more information about Wiley products, visit www.wiley.com.

Library of Congress Control Number: 2023947361

ISBN: 978-1-394-18688-4 (pbk); ISBN 978-1-394-18690-7 (ebk); ISBN 978-1-394-18689-1 (ebk)

SKY10057765_101723

Contents at a Glance

Table of Contents

Introduction

wrote this book because I take care of women every day. I see women in my medical office daily from young teenagers to women in their 90s, and the women who have always seemed most surprised and unprepared for the many physical and emotional changes suddenly causing great disruption to their lives are women in the throes of perimenopause.

It seems there are books, and YouTube channels, and podcasts and websites for women who would like to be pregnant, those who *are* pregnant, women who are parents, and young professionals, and even guides for living your best life as a senior citizen. But there is an information desert when it comes to explaining, preparing for, and treating the issues of women who find themselves in the years in between reproductive life and their menopausal years.

Perimenopause can last up to ten years, and the one line I have heard from my patients more times than I can count, is "Why didn't anyone ever tell me that this was going to happen?"

Perimenopause is almost always a complicated mix of seemingly random physical and emotional signs and symptoms in need of attention and explanation. I have heard the following (sometimes all in one day):

>> "I think I'm going crazy."

>> "My hormones must be all out of whack."

>> "I cannot get out of bed."

>> "I have suddenly gained 15 pounds overnight."

>> "I'm in a bad mood all the time."

>> "I can't concentrate, and I have constant brain fog."

This truly is a time where you can be unlucky enough to have many of the well-known menopausal symptoms like hot flashes, night sweats, low energy, poor sleep, vaginal dryness, and irritable bladder, and at the very same time suffer from heavy and irregular periods that remind you of your teenage years. It's a lot to deal with, and the lack of preparation and available information makes it worse!

Of course, it's not all about the hormones. Lifestyle and general health habits have a huge effect on how you may manage during the perimenopausal transition years. Your ability to deal with stress, your diet, and exercise habits all affect your health as you move through midlife and into your menopausal years. I have lots of information in this book about all these aspects of the perimenopause transition as well, because a plan should include a look at all the components of health and well-being. There are so many companies that claim that if you just buy their vitamins, supplements, or detox regimens you will slow down (or stop!) the aging process and all your symptoms will go away. Sometimes you may begin to think they may be worth a try, because the information on safe, evidence-based solutions may be hard to find, and doctors who have the knowledge and the ability to share that information with you seem like a rarity.

I am hoping that this book can fill in some of the missing pieces. I am hoping you can use this book as a guide; choose the topics and the chapters that seem to have the information you've been looking for; arm yourself with facts and data and details that you can use to bring up difficult topics with your own doctor. I have tried to provide enough information for you to be able to make informed decisions about your health and talk to a medical provider who will truly be your partner during this difficult time.

About This Book

This book is not written to sell you anything; it's not to judge what you may feel comfortable with or what you may choose as your plan for going through your perimenopausal transition. Some women feel that they need to "tough it out" and some feel that taking a medication or seeing a therapist is "giving in" or "giving up." I want you to live your best, most comfortable and healthiest life as you move through your 30s, 40s and 50s. This book is written to provide you with lots of evidence and science-based information so that you can make informed and sensible decisions on how to best care for yourself at this time. I cover the questions that many of my patients ask me, focusing on topics that come up so frequently in my office visits with midlife women. Whether you are just starting to go through this transition or are on the threshold of menopause, you will find lots of information about health and well-being. You can read and re-read and tuck this information away for use at whatever time seems most appropriate in your perimenopausal years.

Foolish Assumptions

Every author must make a few assumptions about her audience, and I've made a few assumptions about you.

>> You're a woman.

>> You want to understand the changes that are happening in your body and mind.

>> You want clear, science-based but easy-to-understand explanations.

>> You would like to know what your risks are for certain diseases and medical illnesses as you age and how you can lower your risk.

>> You want to be able to make choices from various safe treatment alternatives.

>> You would like to have information that will enable you to have an informed discussion with a medical professional and make decisions together about options.

>> You read books.

If this sounds like you, welcome to *Perimenopause for Dummies*.

Icons Used in This Book

Here and there, sprinkled in the margins of the book, you'll find little pictures that point to important parts of the text. Here are the icons we use and what they mean.

These little nuggets of advice can save you valuable time or prevent headaches in the future. It's sage advice from teachers who have already suffered the slings and arrows of bad decisions.

Think of these warnings as little flags that a minesweeper has placed in the field before you so you know where you can safely step and where you definitely can't.

File these things away in your mind because, somewhere down the road, you'll be glad you did.

Text marked with a Technical Stuff icon is interesting, but ultimately it isn't essential for getting a handle on perimenopause. If you want to get in and get out, you can skip these bits without compromising your understanding of the topic.

Beyond the Book

In addition to the pages you're reading right now, this book comes with a free, access-anywhere online Cheat Sheet that summarizes some of our key advice at a glance. To access this Cheat Sheet, go to www.dummies.com, and type **Perimenopause** in the search box.

Where to Go from Here

If you want a complete picture of perimenopause, you can definitely read this book straight through. But you don't have to go cover to cover to meet your needs.

For information on what's going on with your menstrual cycle or hormonal shifts in general, head to Part 2. If you want to understand changes that may be occurring in your sleep patterns, or if you're experiencing symptoms like brain fog, skip ahead to Part 3. Looking for some tips on diet or exercise? You can find that in Part 4.

However you read it, this book is intended to serve you and help provide you the information you need to navigate perimenopause and all its changes in good spirits and good health.

1

The Facts of Life at Perimenopause

IN THIS CHAPTER

» Understanding what perimenopause is

» Knowing the symptoms of perimenopause

» Recognizing the difference between perimenopause and other conditions

» Preparing for the physical changes

» Consulting with a trusted medical professional

Chapter **1**

Welcome to Perimenopause

For women, it seems like life is all about stages. You have the childhood stage, which somehow ends around puberty, when things change and start to take a more serious turn. Then you have the reproductive stage, governed by hormonal cycles, during which the usual goals are to avoid pregnancies or to create pregnancies; also to feel well and stable emotionally. Jump over quite a few years, and you have a non-reproductive stage called menopause, when the ovaries completely shut down, all hormone levels are low, and keeping healthy and living a full life are the usual objectives.

But what about that huge gap of time between those reproductive years and the menopausal ones? You have a decade (or so) where you may still worry about a pregnancy (or you may still try to achieve one), where you experience symptoms that appear when your hormones vary widely from week to week, and even from day to day.

During these years, you may find yourself dealing with brain fog, vaginal dryness, insomnia, mood swings, and low energy at the same time that you find yourself with heavy and irregular vaginal bleeding. For these years, I'm guessing that no one ever sat you down and said, "This is what may happen between age 38 and 53." That's what this book is about. Welcome to perimenopause!

To get started, this chapter offers a brief overview of what causes various perimenopausal changes at this time of your life, as well as what symptoms you may have and why. You can dive deeper into all the topics mentioned here by looking into the chapters that deal specifically with each subject.

Understanding What Perimenopause Is

Perimenopause is a time, in years, of transition. It involves a move away from the regularity of hormonal release, monthly ovulation, and the menstrual cycle. Hormones cause physical and emotional changes in your body, and the more regularly your body releases these hormones, the more stable you feel. When both ovulation and hormone release start to become irregular, you've entered perimenopause. In general, perimenopause can start for a woman anywhere over the age of 35 and last until about age 53. (The average age of menopause is about 51.)

Between 35 and 53 years old is a very wide range, and I don't mean everyone experiences perimenopause from the age of 35 to 53. When you start perimenopause sometimes depends on how regularly your body released hormones in your 20s and 30s. (See Chapter 6 for more on that topic.) For most women, irregularities in menstrual cycles are just one of the signs that perimenopause is approaching. Swings in moods, lack of concentration, poor energy, weight gain, and insomnia are some of the other hallmarks of aging out of your reproductive years and entering the perimenopausal transition.

PERIMENOPAUSE AND WOMEN OF COLOR

An August 23, 2023, article in the *New York Times* entitled "How Menopause Affects Women of Color" reviewed the ways in which the experience of perimenopause and menopause is different in various communities. The article notes that researchers who followed a group of more than 3,000 women during perimenopause and menopause have found a few key differences: Black and Hispanic women reach menopause earlier than white, Chinese, and Japanese women, and sometimes with more severe symptoms. Black women are more likely to experience more intense and frequent hot flashes, and endure them for more years, than women of other races. So Black women may generally start their transition earlier, and if a Black woman begins experiencing symptoms even in her 30s that sound like perimenopause, those symptoms certainly warrant a medical evaluation.

Because of racial disparities in the healthcare system, often when women of color seek care, they may encounter physicians who "aren't fully equipped to help them navigate that transition," according to the *New York Times* article.

Several studies have found that when women of color do find a menopause specialist, that specialist is less likely to provide them with a prescription for hormone therapy, as compared to white patients. This discrepancy in prescription writing may occur because of an unconscious racial bias that leads physicians to believe that a patient's symptoms don't warrant treatment. Untreated hot flashes can lead to an increase in cardiovascular disease; this potential for disease may mean that the undertreatment of women of color may lead to more severe long-term negative health outcomes while they go through their perimenopausal and menopausal years.

Common Perimenopausal Symptoms

You can potentially attribute a laundry list of symptoms to the sudden drop in estrogen levels in your body, along with other hormonal changes that occur in perimenopause. You may not experience all of these symptoms, but if you have just a few (or sometimes even just one), we usually can assume that the hormonal changes of perimenopause are responsible. Here are the common perimenopause symptoms to watch out for:

>> **Interrupted sleep:** The hormones estrogen and neurotransmitter serotonin act as partners in assisting deep, restful sleep; if your body doesn't produce one of these hormones, it also may not stimulate the other.

>> **Hot flashes:** A sudden drop in estrogen levels triggers a *hot flash,* a temporary rise in body temperature, enough to cause sweating and flushing of the face and usually the upper body.

>> **Heart palpitations:** A sudden change in estrogen levels can cause heart flutters because of the hormone adrenaline that your body can release in response to changing hormone levels.

>> **Changes in your menstrual cycle:** Although you can't blame all menstrual irregularities on perimenopause, women commonly start to see irregular bleeding, bleeding between periods, or changes in their bleeding pattern during perimenopause.

>> **Irritability, anxiety, and mood changes:** Often, hormonal swings can result in changes to your mood; premenstrual mood changes can now seem to occur all month long or randomly throughout the cycle.

>> **Brain fog and lack of concentration:** Estrogen plays a role in memory and mental clarity, and changes in estrogen levels (along with poor sleep) can cause changes in cognitive function.

>> **Vaginal and genital discomfort:** Because the vagina has many estrogen receptors, the vagina stays healthy when the body has estrogen, especially in the genital area. Women often see the result of a decrease in their estrogen levels when intercourse becomes painful.

>> **Urinary changes:** A decrease in estrogen levels may lead to increased frequency or irritability of the bladder; bladder issues may also relate to changes in vaginal health because the vagina and the *urethra* (the endpoint of the urinary system) are so close together.

>> **Skin changes:** Lower estrogen levels cause your skin to lose firmness and elasticity. Without estrogen, skin often becomes thin, loose, and droopy. You may notice hair loss and other skin changes, as well.

Although medical science doesn't yet have a way to definitively attribute these symptoms to perimenopause, knowing that almost every perimenopausal woman has these symptoms at one time or another during her transition to menopause may make you feel a little less disturbed by the ones happening to you.

While you make your way through this book and consult with your doctor about various signs and symptoms that are causing a decrease in the quality of your life, remember that just because women commonly experience these symptoms during perimenopause doesn't mean that you can't do anything about them.

NEVER HESITATE TO TALK TO YOUR DOCTOR!

It's important when reading about perimenopause, in this book or elsewhere, to keep in mind that every woman experiences this stage — in terms of symptoms and their severity as well as age and other factors differently. Don't wait until your timeline or symptoms exactly match a checklist in your head to talk to your doctor.

Here's an example from my practice (I share more in Chapter 19): A 52-year-old lady came to see me for her annual exam. One year before, she had still been having monthly periods and no perimenopausal symptoms. Her diet was healthy, she was regularly exercising, and she felt emotionally well.

One year later, she reported to me that since that last visit, her periods had spaced out, appearing now once every four to five months. For the entire year since her last visit, she had been sleeping poorly, having mood swings, and feeling irritable a lot of the time. I asked why she waited all 12 months to come back to see me, and she said she thought I couldn't do anything to help her because she hadn't gone a full 12 months without a period!

After talking about all the ways that I possibly could help her, we chose a vaginal contraceptive ring. This is the lowest dose combination contraceptive, and she wouldn't have to remember to take something every day; it would likely relieve her symptoms, regulate her bleeding, and improve her overall mood (if hot flashes, which caused her to wake up at night, led to the irritability and poor sleep).

Knowing if It's Perimenopause or Something Else

It can be easy to attribute symptoms such as depression or sleep problems, weight gain, or heart palpitations as clear signals of perimenopause, but this can also be a dangerous assumption for individuals and indeed medical professionals to make.

If you suspect something is going on that is more than perimenopause, it's important to express your concerns (and symptoms) to your doctor. You can put your health at great risk by ignoring symptoms or writing them off as inevitable or untreatable or "just" perimenopause.

Sometimes what seems like a symptom of perimenopause could be caused by something else; you and your doctor need to rule out other, serious medical conditions before treating what seems like a symptom of perimenopause.

WARNING

Anytime that you start having symptoms that confuse you or that seem new and different, have your doctor or medical professional evaluate you. Don't self-treat, and don't rely on questionable information from people who don't realize the medical implications of treating your conditions without an evaluation.

Evaluating the causes of your symptoms

Because medical symptoms and conditions can appear in the perimenopausal years and may masquerade as perimenopausal symptoms, discuss them with your doctor, who can evaluate them so that you both know you have the right treatment plan and you haven't missed anything.

Sleep problems

Interrupted sleep can be caused by poor sleep hygiene, which can include

>> Watching computer or TV screens before bed

>> Taking certain medications

>> Drinking alcohol

>> Smoking

>> Dealing with mental conditions such as anxiety and depression

>> Suffering from pain conditions or headaches

If you experience any of the medical conditions in the preceding list for the first time in perimenopause, investigate the cause or causes with your medical provider.

Hot flashes

A lack of estrogen most commonly causes hot flashes, but other conditions can also cause them, such as

>> Thyroid disorders

>> Diabetes

>> High blood pressure

>> Electrolyte imbalances

>> Infections

>> Fevers

>> Anxiety

>> Heart conditions

>> Heat stroke

>> Obesity

Heart palpitations

You can experience heart palpitations because of

>> Various heart conditions

>> Thyroid disorders

- » Pregnancy
- » Gastrointestinal problems
- » Medications
- » Anxiety disorders
- » Pain syndromes
- » Poor sleep

Menstrual cycle irregularity

Changes in your menstrual cycle can occur because of

- » Anatomical problems inside the uterus such as fibroids or polyps
- » Medications
- » Pregnancy
- » Thyroid disorders
- » Infections
- » Pre-cancer or cancerous conditions inside the uterus
- » Trauma

Mood issues

You can find separating irritability, anxiety, and mood changes from true mental health conditions difficult while you go through perimenopause. You may have experienced depression and anxiety before you began your perimenopause transition, or those conditions may have just appeared at this midlife time.

Eliminating all the situational reasons for mood swings can help you check whether these sudden changes result from hormonal changes, situational changes, or true mental health issues that you need to address. A skilled clinician should be able to help you figure it out.

Life events that can lead to mood swings include

- » Changing relationships
- » Illness in family members
- » Job stressors
- » Children leaving home or returning home

Mental focus issues

Brain fog, lack of mental clarity, and poor concentration can have many different causes:

>> Medications

>> Mental health conditions

>> Stress

>> Thyroid conditions

>> Alcohol, tobacco, or drug use

>> Brain tumors

>> Neurological conditions

>> Vascular damage

>> Stroke

>> Heart conditions

All of these factors can cause you to have difficulty remembering or thinking. Although estrogen levels can affect clarity of thinking, the human body needs many different hormones to support healthy brain function.

Vaginal discomfort

You can experience vaginal and genital discomfort for a number of reasons:

>> Infections

>> Trauma

>> Pelvic floor weakness or relaxation

>> Lack of tissue elasticity

>> Certain neurological conditions

>> Skin conditions

If you had vaginal comfort until the time of midlife and then started to have dryness in the vaginal area, which led to painful intercourse, you can usually rule out these other conditions, and your doctor and you can consider vaginal estrogen or moisturizer treatments.

Urinary changes

You may experience urinary changes for a number of reasons:

>> Infections

>> Neurological conditions

>> Bladder damage

>> Medications

>> Childbirth

>> Mental conditions

Your doctor and you need to assess these factors, rather than just assuming that your urinary issues come from the normal changes of perimenopause.

Skin changes

Although skin changes commonly occur during perimenopause, those changes can have a variety of causes that your doctor and you should consider:

>> Years of sun exposure

>> Pre-cancerous or cancerous changes on the skin

>> Skin conditions caused by auto-immune diseases

REMEMBER

Estrogen applied to the skin hasn't been shown to improve skin changes caused by aging.

Talking about your symptoms

Perimenopause can be a significant turning point in life, one in which your body and mind undergoes shifts that can be profound. Beyond physical symptoms, perimenopause comes at a time in life where you might be seeing change in your life circumstances, as well — at home or at work, for example.

Sharing experiences, symptoms, and emotions is more than just chit chat — for many women, it can be a lifeline. Sharing what you are going through with others can help you (and them) understand and better navigate this stage.

Talking to others in the same boat

As a woman experiencing perimenopause, you need to take care of yourself and get support from people who understand your situation. You usually can find women in similar situations, experiencing similar symptoms, without looking too far. Friends, relatives, or coworkers within a few years of your age can likely provide good support when you want to discuss your symptoms.

Support groups — in person or on social media — can also provide places to find what you need. You may even get recommendations to a doctor or other specialized healthcare practitioner through these support systems. (See Appendix B for information about these support groups.)

WARNING

However, please don't confuse your online search with medical expertise. You can stumble upon so much misinformation that you can't easily differentiate the real medical information from the scammers.

Talking with your partner about perimenopause symptoms

Just at the time that your kids move out (if you have them), or at least have their own fish to fry, and you have more time to spend romantically with your partner, your moods become erratic, your body becomes unwilling, and your libido disappears. Although interest in and capacity for sex doesn't automatically decline in this midlife stage, you may need to do a lot more work to keep things happy and healthy in the sex department.

Some women in their 40s are still interested in fertility — and you just can't close things down sexually if that's where your heart lies.

When it comes to all these changes occurring in perimenopause, let your partner in on exactly what's happening and what you're feeling.

Let them know that your hormones are changing, which influences your interest. Come up with ideas together that can get the spark going for both of you:

>> Set a date on the calendar.

>> Go to a special place that has sparked your romantic feelings in the past.

>> Try different activities in the bedroom (or living room, or wherever).

>> Use more lubrication.

>> Give a different position a try.

>> Find a way to destress.

Whatever you need, don't keep it to yourself.

REMEMBER

Many relationships have been ruined by the lack of communication and understanding that happens in this phase of life. Sometimes, a woman in perimenopause doesn't understand her own body's changes, let alone expect her partner to understand them and adjust behavior accordingly. Your relationship can evolve to a new level of meaning and pleasure.

The Physical Changes in Perimenopause

Despite what people think, no studies link perimenopause with a major change in metabolism, and perimenopause doesn't, in and of itself, lead to weight gain. Although the hormonal changes of perimenopause alone don't cause weight gain, perimenopausal and menopausal women do tend to gain weight while they age. (Studies have shown about a 1- to 2-pound gain per year.)

Weight redistributes and starts to accumulate around the middle, and you also start to lose muscle mass. To keep these two things from happening, you have to monitor the type and volume of food that you eat. (See Chapter 13 for discussion of healthy eating in perimenopause.)

You have many ways to lose weight and to build muscle; whichever method you choose must be one that fits into your schedule consistently, includes enough fiber and protein, and hopefully includes an activity that you enjoy. Being overweight or obese in perimenopause, where fat accumulates around your middle and stays there, has many health implications. This extra fat increases your risk of

>> Heart disease and stroke

>> Diabetes

>> Vascular disease

>> High cholesterol

Calling in the Professionals

If you're in your 40s or early 50s and experiencing the symptoms listed in the section "Common perimenopausal symptoms," earlier in this chapter, you're probably in perimenopause. If you think that's the case, make an appointment with your medical practitioner to get your symptoms evaluated.

As I discuss in the section "Evaluating the causes of your symptoms," earlier in this chapter, not all symptoms that feel like perimenopause actually are caused by perimenopause. Before deciding on treatment, your doctor and you need to rule out other medical conditions. Your practitioner can help you deal with the undesirable symptoms of perimenopause while helping you prevent serious health conditions.

After a year goes by without a period, or you determine in some way that your ovaries are no longer functioning, you're officially in menopause, where you'll spend the rest of your life.

With some self-assessment and a bit of determination — as well as the information you can find in this book — you can reduce troublesome perimenopausal symptoms, prevent disease, and promote a long and healthy life.

Chapter **2**

Getting Acquainted with Your Midlife Body

You may be noticing some (or even many) physical and emotional changes, all of which typically occur while you begin your transition to menopause. Although every woman experiences different changes at varying levels of intensity, some symptoms are standard among most women.

You probably expect some of these symptoms, and some symptoms may take you by surprise. Anticipating these changes and knowing when (or if) you can or should intervene can put you ahead in the perimenopause game.

Although I hope that all women will experience perimenopause and menopause itself with as little disruption or discomfort as possible, anticipating what you *may* experience during this stage can help you navigate it with more ease, self-compassion, and sometimes even humor. In this chapter, I walk through these changes as a sort of overview.

Identifying Physical Changes of the Midlife Body

Have you ever had the experience of passing by a store window or a full-length mirror, looking at the reflection, and saying, "Who is *that*?" You see someone that you don't recognize — and usually not in a complimentary way. Seemingly overnight, serious changes have taken place in your body.

Gaining weight and redistributing body fat

One of the most common physical complaints of women reaching the perimenopause stage of life is weight gain. Not just a few pounds of weight gain everywhere, but specifically a substantial amount of belly fat: extra girth that seemingly appeared overnight and parked itself right around your middle. Even if you never had belly fat before, your diet hasn't changed, and you do endless sit-ups and abdominal crunches throughout the day, it seems impossible to get rid of your spare tire. Is it inevitable?

The hormonal changes of midlife might make you more likely to gain weight around your abdomen than around your hips and thighs. This type of weight gain may also relate to genetic factors (look at the fat distribution of the other women in your family) and to lifestyle and aging.

Weight gain around the middle increases the risk for heart disease, diabetes, and breathing problems, among other medical conditions, so it makes sense to try to prevent this annoying accumulation of fat.

Disappearing muscles

Muscle mass typically diminishes with age, while fat increases. Losing muscle mass slows the rate at which your body uses calories. This slows down your metabolism and makes it more challenging to maintain a healthy weight. You may start to feel that your body is sagging in areas that used to be muscular. Hormonal changes and a lack of regular physical activity are associated with a decrease in muscle mass and strength.

TIP

Increased physical activity, including resistance training, can help maintain your metabolism and help prevent this loss of muscle.

Changing heart health, blood pressure, and cholesterol

Women are generally protected from heart disease while they're in their young reproductive years because of the effect that estrogen has on both the heart and the blood vessels. When estrogen starts to diminish around the time of perimenopause, so does its protective effect on the heart. Between age 45 and 65, men experience three times more heart attacks than women. But after age 65, women have more heart attacks than men.

WARNING

Menopausal women are at an increased risk for heart attacks, but heart disease can start much earlier. The perimenopausal years are a good time to look at your risk factors for heart disease and heart attacks, and try to modify any risk factors that you can.

High blood pressure is one risk factor for heart disease and is more likely to occur while you get older. Typically, women's blood pressure readings start to rise when their estrogen levels decline, and blood pressure continues to go up through midlife and into menopause. High blood pressure occurs when your heart is trying to pump the blood that's circulating in your body through blood vessels that become narrower while you age. The heart is a pump, and the harder it must work to pump blood through narrow blood vessels, the higher your blood pressure goes.

Blood vessels can also become blocked or narrowed due to the accumulation of cholesterol, also called *plaque*, in those vessels. *Cholesterol* is a fatty substance produced by your liver and also found in certain foods. Your body needs cholesterol to digest food, make hormones, and build cells, among other things. But your doctor probably talks to you a lot about keeping your cholesterol numbers low. Although the body uses cholesterol to build and repair cells, as well as to make certain hormones, too much cholesterol can contribute to blocking blood vessels, leading to high blood pressure and heart disease.

Cholesterol travels through the bloodstream and attaches to the inside of your blood vessels, causing blockages. When you eat too much food that contains cholesterol, the excess intake prompts the liver to make more cholesterol than the body needs. Although genetics play a role in your cholesterol numbers, perimenopause is a great time to adopt a diet and exercise plan to keep your cholesterol in the normal range and decrease your risk while you move toward menopause.

Battling Bone Loss

When you were young, growing and movement were two parts of life that you just took for granted. Bones grew longer and thicker, you got taller, and until about age 30 (except for incidents of trauma), you could run, dance, and jump with little worry about your bones breaking. However, in your perimenopause years, your bones can start to get thin while the amount of new bone being built slows down. If your bones were healthy when you were young (mostly due to a good diet, healthy exercise, and genetics), then at midlife, you don't need to worry too much about them. Perimenopause is the chance to keep those bones strong.

The bladder that betrays you

The first time it happens, it may shock you: that unexpected and uncontrollable dribble. It may happen when you're taking a long walk; it may happen when you've just gotten up from the toilet, thinking you were done; and it may happen when you lift a heavy suitcase to put it on the airport conveyor belt. *Was that urine?*

In your midlife years, you may start to realize that something you always had control over is not so much in your control anymore: your bladder. Lower levels of estrogen make the muscle fibers around the bladder and the *urethra* (the tube that transports urine from the bladder to the outside of your body) less flexible. Estrogen helps increase the healthy muscle tone in that area, which helps prevent leakage. Not all leakage is the same, and leaks are most definitely not inevitable.

PERIMENOPAUSE AND OSTEOPOROSIS

Osteoporosis is a condition where bones become weak and brittle; this condition makes those bones more at risk of breaking. About 25 million Americans have osteoporosis, most of them women. In perimenopause, most women begin losing bone at a rate of 1 percent a year.

Osteoporosis is caused by calcium deficiency in the bones, and estrogen helps get calcium into the bones to prevent osteoporosis. After estrogen levels begin to decrease, as in perimenopause, the body is less efficient at moving calcium into the bones, so those bones get thinner and weaker.

Other things can influence the pathway to osteoporosis, such as genetics, a deficiency of vitamins or minerals, lifestyle habits (smoking and alcohol use), and low activity levels. You can correct many of these things in perimenopause, before the bones start to thin, to improve bone density and slow bone loss.

Risk factors for urinary leakage include

>> Age

>> Poor muscle tone

>> Obesity

>> A history of vaginal deliveries that included long pushing phases or delivering big babies

>> Frequent urinary tract infections

>> A lack of estrogen in the vaginal area

>> Damage to the tissues around the urethra from trauma

There are different kinds of urinary incontinence:

>> **Stress incontinence:** When urine leaks if you laugh, cough, sneeze, or lift something heavy. These actions cause an increase in pressure in the abdomen, which causes the urethra to involuntarily open a bit, causing leakage. Because this leakage is a problem of anatomy, it requires an anatomical solution, such as exercise, physical therapy, or surgery.

>> **Urge incontinence:** Less common, but associated with a strong urgency to urinate, accompanied by some leakage even before the bathroom is reached. It may cause you to get up multiple times at night to urinate. Overactive nerves to the bladder lead to this type of incontinence, and your doctor can treat it with various medications or nerve stimulation devices.

>> **Mixed incontinence:** Elements of both stress and urge incontinence. You may leak randomly, get up at night, and also leak when coughing or laughing hard.

Leakage because of a urinary tract infection or an irritative bladder condition called *interstitial cystitis* can also occur. These conditions do tend to occur more frequently in the perimenopausal and menopausal years. To determine the proper treatment, you need to have a discussion with your healthcare provider, who conducts a bladder evaluation and can then diagnose your urinary issues.

Dry skin and hair distribution changes

You may have noticed that your skin has gotten drier over the years. The medical community thinks that diminishing hormone levels play at least a part in skin becoming drier, although some women just have drier skin from a very young age. You may also notice that the hair on the top of your head, where it belongs, is starting to become thin, while hair in places where it doesn't belong (such as on your chin) is starting to appear regularly and rapidly.

A patient came to see me for a hormone consultation visit. I saw on my schedule that she was 48 years old and new to my practice. When she sat down and I started my usual list of questions, she answered me with, "No, I don't have any hot flashes or night sweats. I want estrogen cream so that I can rub it on my skin — it's so dry and thin, and I've tried everything!" Unfortunately, I had to tell her that's not the way it works.

Unfortunately, no medical evidence suggests that rubbing estrogen on thinning skin can make it more moist, thick, or wrinkle free. The bottom line is that during perimenopause, the skin loses some of its elasticity and tightness, and it becomes thinner and saggier.

The skin changes that you see may include more laugh lines, also called crow's feet, around your eyes and mouth, thinning of the skin on the back of your hands, and bruises that develop more easily on your legs. Some of these changes may occur because of aging skin, sun damage, and exposure, but some of these issues can occur because of the diminishing levels of estrogen that accompany perimenopause.

Collagen and *elastin* (proteins found in the connective tissue of the skin) are responsible for plumping up the cheeks and areas around the eyes, as well as the skin on the back of the hands and all over the body. Lower estrogen levels decrease the amount of collagen and elastin in your skin. Other things that can decrease these proteins include sun exposure, smoking, and a high-sugar diet. When the skin and the layers underneath the skin lose their flexibility, you see a loss of firmness and smoothness to skin all over.

Hair loss can happen while you age because hair follicles are very receptive to hormones. Female hormones, such as estrogen, are in abundance in your young, reproductive years, but their production starts to slow down in perimenopause. The female body also produces low levels of male hormones during reproductive years, and these male hormones are still present in perimenopause. The estrogen levels start to diminish, but the hair follicles continue to be affected by the male hormones (called *androgens* — more on these later in this chapter), and hair follicles respond by allowing the hair to fall out. The androgens can also affect hair follicles by shrinking them.

Also, hair goes through natural cycles of loss and replacement. Androgens shorten the natural cycle of hair loss and replacement, creating a longer period time of during which hair falls out and a shorter period of time during which the follicle creates new hair.

Other factors influence hair loss: thyroid function, genetics, diet, autoimmune diseases, medications, stress, and chemotherapy. Your healthcare provider can prescribe medications that can help slow down hair loss, but giving such a prescription requires the doctor to do a thorough evaluation, including bloodwork, to look for causes.

Hair showing up in places such as the chin and chest also gives you a sign of an increasing influence of male-associated hormones. Most women find some way to remove these stray hairs — by plucking or using electrolysis or hair-removal creams. The presence of these stray hairs usually doesn't indicate a worrisome medical condition unless accompanied by other symptoms, such as severe headaches, unusual menstrual bleeding patterns, or pigmented skin (which can all be signs of disorders of the endocrine system).

Changes in the vagina and vulva

Every woman has a different relationship with her genital area. Maybe you've been comfortable your whole life looking at yourself down there, touching the anatomy, familiarizing yourself with the skin, the folds, the parts that have always been yours. You feel comfortable putting a tampon in your vagina and shaving or waxing your vulva. And you know when something feels not right.

Or maybe you haven't explored. You may not have used tampons and may not feel comfortable looking at or touching the various parts of your genital region. Figure 2-1 gives you a very general anatomical drawing of this region so that, while I discuss parts of your body that might be changing, you have some idea of what I'm talking about.

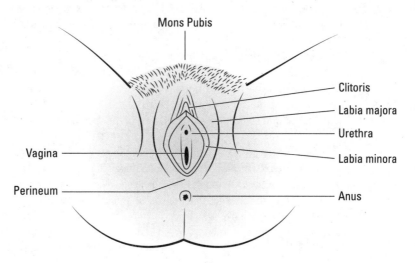

FIGURE 2-1: The vagina and vulva.

After you start perimenopause, you may notice that the external area, like the rest of your skin, tends to lose some of its plumpness. The tissues may become thin and dry. Some women experience irritation, itching, pain, or burning. Some may feel that, at the time of sexual activity, their body doesn't produce as much natural lubrication as it used to.

In truth, estrogen is the vagina's best friend. When estrogen levels start to fluctuate, and then to diminish while you go through your perimenopause years and into menopause, a lack of estrogen affects the vaginal and vulvar tissues. They can become drier and thinner, have less natural lubrication and comfort, and tear more easily. This change may make penetrative sex uncomfortable, or at the worst, impossible. If you do experience any of these discomforts, you can discuss the many treatments available with your doctor. (I talk about some of these treatments in Chapter 7.)

TIP

If your doctor doesn't bring up this conversation at your visit, talk to them about your specific symptoms and discomforts so that they can recommend appropriate treatments. If your doctor doesn't offer you any recommendations (or if they say, "This is just something to be expected"), find a different practitioner or inquire about some of the suggestions in this book (see Chapter 7 for my advice about how to keep the vagina and vulva healthy and pain free throughout perimenopause and menopause).

OUT WITH THE OLD (TERMINOLOGY) — GOOD RIDDANCE

Vaginal atrophy is the terrible medical term that was coined to describe what happens to the vagina after the body's estrogen levels start to diminish. Sounds like a vagina that's going to shrivel up and disappear, doesn't it? We now (after years of advocacy meetings) use the term *Genitourinary Syndrome of Menopause* (GSM), as an all-inclusive term to describe the many symptoms that are associated with a lack of estrogen to the genital area, including vaginal dryness, burning and discharge, itching, urinary urgency, recurrent urinary tract infections, discomfort with intercourse, decreased lubrication during sexual activity, and shortening and tightening of the vaginal canal and tissues.

Sometimes, the best way to prevent or to slow the progress of GSM is to have regular sexual activity, which increases circulation to the genital area and promotes natural lubrication and elasticity to the tissues. However, to use this advice successfully, you must be aware of the changes that may occur and have a plan of action to intervene before these changes make sexual activity difficult. I go over how your sex life may change after you start perimenopause in Chapter 7.

Understanding Hormonal Changes in Perimenopause

Everyone knows something about hormones. You probably know that they're some kind of chemical messengers that your body makes, and they're responsible for things. But what things? You may be a little confused about the details.

Back when you were in middle school, sometimes later (and sometimes never), some adult in your life may have given you The Talk. A basic explanation about how women have ovaries, and ovaries produce eggs, and you need eggs to make babies — sort of making it sound like you have ovaries only so that you can procreate.

But the ideal talk explains so much more than ovaries as tools of baby-making. It explains how several organs in the body are responsible for making hormones, this hormone production changes throughout your life, and those changes will result in symptoms that you may experience, depending on your age and your history. This talk helps you prepare for those changes. When you can anticipate and know what's coming, you can much better prepare than if you're surprised by the hormonal changes to your body and mind that you'll probably encounter.

Although this book focuses on the changes to anticipate during perimenopause, to properly understand that phase, you need to review (or maybe realize for the first time) what happens with a woman's hormones before the age of perimenopause. Before midlife and before you start to feel the effects of changes in your hormone production, what's happening while your body makes all the hormones of reproduction?

Only one of the major functions of hormones, specifically sex hormones (estrogen, progesterone, and testosterone), is to prepare the body to produce life. A typical menstrual cycle is approximately 28 days (although it can be longer or shorter) and involves the following phases:

» **Follicular phase:** Starts from Day 1 of menstrual bleeding. In the first few days of the cycle, the brain triggers the ovaries to produce estrogen. This estrogen (among other things) helps a lining to build up within the uterus. This lining consists of blood and tissue, and it thickens the inside cavity of the uterus, called the *endometrium*.

» **Ovulation:** About halfway through the cycle, or about Day 14, the ovary releases an egg (a process called *ovulation*) in response to another chemical trigger from the brain.

>> **Luteal phase:** After ovulation, estrogen levels drop a bit, but progesterone levels increase. This change in hormone levels stabilizes that thick endometrial lining in case the egg is fertilized and needs to be implanted in that lining.

>> **Menstruation:** If no fertilized egg attaches to the endometrium (meaning no pregnancy), the uterus doesn't need the thick uterine lining, so that lining sheds in response to the drop in estrogen and progesterone levels.

This cycle repeats itself approximately every 28 days if the ovaries continue to release eggs.

After age 35, and certainly after age 40, most women have a change in their hormone production, related mostly to a change in ovulation. Releasing eggs may continue to occur monthly, but more often, ovulation will become irregular. The other *stimulation triggers* (signals from the brain to the ovaries) continue: The ovaries still produce estrogen in response to a signal from the brain. A lining still builds up in the uterus in response to that estrogen production.

But wait! If you don't ovulate (or if the ovulation occurs sooner or later than expected), then the hormonal changes that start to occur are caused by a change in the amount or the timing of the progesterone production. Without progesterone, that endometrial lining isn't stable and doesn't have an exact trigger telling it when to shed. It may shed earlier than expected, later than expected, or not at all. (See Chapter 5 for more on bleeding patterns.)

This lack of regular, cyclic progesterone production causes many of the irregular bleeding patterns that start to occur in perimenopause, as well as the emotional ups and downs, disrupted sleep, and lack of mental focus. While perimenopause progresses, estrogen production may change as well; the ovaries become less able to respond to the stimulation from the brain, and estrogen production in the ovaries begins to become irregular.

You may feel great during some months (or weeks) when the ovaries respond to all the right stimulation from the brain and make estrogen and progesterone at the proper times of the month within the menstrual cycle. But sometimes, none of the signals or the responses occur the way that they're supposed to, which can cause you to swing from low to high hormone production, then high to low, with your symptoms swinging up and down while your body responds to these drastic hormonal changes. Just like in puberty.

The Disappearing, Reappearing, and Surprising Period

Because the definition of *menopause* is 12 consecutive months without a period, usually anything that doesn't meet that definition isn't considered menopause. During perimenopause, you may have many of the symptoms that we associate with menopause, such as hot flashes, irritability, mood swings, poor sleep, and vaginal dryness — but you can also still get your period. Yay.

WARNING

You may have the lovely experience of counting down the days during which you have no bleeding, getting to 10 months in a row — and then suddenly (and usually on vacation), your period returns in all of its heavy, clotty, unexpected glory. You're still in perimenopause.

You may be lucky enough to have a monthly period like clockwork, never really experiencing an irregular perimenopausal bleeding pattern. But then 12 months go by with no period. When you hit that 12th dry month, by definition, you're in menopause.

More likely, you'll have a bleeding pattern that falls somewhere in between these two extremes. Bleeding and periods are likely to be irregular, skipping here and there, becoming heavier and lighter — and this pattern can go on for months or years leading up to menopause.

TIP

Do you have to endure this annoying pattern if it interferes with your quality of life (and your ability to wear white pants)? Absolutely not. (Please see Chapter 5, where I talk about various ways to deal with irregular bleeding patterns that interfere with your quality of life.)

REMEMBER

Here's an important medical rule: If you go 12 months without a period, and therefore meet the definition of menopause (assuming something such as medication, cancer, or surgery doesn't cause the lack of a period), and then your period seems to come back, that bleed isn't actually a period. It's called *post-menopausal bleeding*, and you should have it evaluated by your healthcare provider.

A patient came to see me because she was *sure* she was in menopause. She was 46 years old and hadn't had a period in four months. She was having night sweats, low energy, and mood swings. Before having a conversation about treating her menopausal symptoms, we did a pregnancy test: And it was positive! After some of the shock wore off, we did an ultrasound, and she was exactly three months pregnant. Whether you see a pregnancy at this stage of your life as a happy or stressful event, this is *not* something to find out by surprise.

FEARING (OR HOPING FOR) PREGNANCY

WARNING

Plenty of women are pursuing fertility and pregnancy after age 40. Whether it's a case of waiting for the right time, the right partner, or financial stability, or because of a change of heart, over 100,000 women over the age of 40 give birth every year in the United States.

When periods become irregular, that's a sign that ovulations may also become irregular, which makes fertility a little harder to track. If you don't know when or if you ovulate, you also don't know what the chances are that you may become pregnant.

Even if you're having only a few periods a year, don't mistake that pattern for a confirmation that you can't get pregnant. If you're sexually active, in perimenopause, and don't want a pregnancy, please consider some form of birth control.

Your doctor may offer to prescribe you hormonal birth control to prevent pregnancy while also relieving some bothersome perimenopausal symptoms, or they may suggest non-hormonal methods of birth control, such as condoms or a copper IUD. (See more on birth control options in Chapter 6.)

Dealing with Hormonal Instability

Hormones are (mostly) helpful in your body. Having some type of stability to your body's production of hormones can contribute to a feeling of calm. Stability can come from hormones being produced at regular intervals, where you can anticipate the changes that occur in your normal menstrual cycle. This cycle usually consists of

- **Menstruation:** Bleeding for several days, usually accompanied by good energy, in spite of bleeding. Emotionally, you likely feel well at this time because estrogen levels start to build.

- **Follicular phase:** During the five to ten days leading up to ovulation at mid-cycle, most women also usually experience a sense of calm, high energy, and the clarity of thought associated with higher levels of estrogen.

- **Ovulation:** Occurs in the middle of the 28-day cycle, and you may feel the physical symptoms associated with ovulation: bloating, cramping, and increased discharge.

- **Luteal phase:** Several days after ovulation, premenstrual feelings begin. While hormone levels start to go down, physical and emotional symptoms may appear, such as poor sleep, irritability, poor concentration, and mood swings.

Bleeding begins again — and the whole cycle starts again. Although you might think that many of the symptoms outlined in the preceding bullet list would interfere with your quality of life, the fact that they're predictable and expected can create a sense of balance. They occur again and again, in a monthly and well-known pattern.

Even if not every phase of your normal menstrual cycle feels the same or even feels pleasant, having a regular cycle — with the regular release of estrogen and progesterone at the same (or similar) times of the month so that you can anticipate how you'll feel at various times of the month — can give you a sense of stability and well-being.

REMEMBER

In menopause, you also get a sense of stability. Your body isn't producing or releasing hormones at all, so you can treat whatever symptoms you experience from this phase of life to provide relief. And at least you know what you'll likely feel every day — you usually don't have to deal with unexpected swings or changes.

Estrogen

But the in-between, unstable stage — this perimenopausal stage — can last anywhere from a few months to seven years (or more). During this stage, your body produces estrogen in fits and starts; and estrogen actively helps with so many physical and mental functions, as well as a sense of well-being. This irregular production of estrogen can leave you wondering how you're going to feel from one day to the next, both emotionally and physically.

You'll have days or weeks where your body produces enough estrogen to provide good energy, restful sleep, sharp concentration, better moods, and a better libido. During the days or weeks when estrogen production is on the downswing, you'll experience exactly the opposite: hot flashes, night sweats, irritability, low energy, low libido, vaginal dryness, and brain fog. To make matters worse, these swings can happen daily, weekly, or for some people, even hourly. This instability in hormone production causes the highs and lows of perimenopause.

Progesterone

Progesterone, which the ovaries produce after ovulation, can

>> Promote better and deeper sleep

>> Make some women feel calm

>> Make some women feel lethargic

>> Increase appetite

>> Slow the digestive process, making some women feel full or bloated

When ovulation doesn't occur (or doesn't occur regularly) and progesterone levels remain low, symptoms of premenstrual syndrome (PMS) may appear:

>> Mood swings

>> Irritability

>> Insomnia

>> Depression or anxiety

>> Physical symptoms, such as joint pain and headaches

Women's bodies also produce hormones called *androgens* in relatively small amounts in the ovaries and adrenal glands. These hormones, which include testosterone, trigger sexual desire, help build bone, maintain muscle mass, and bolster energy levels. In perimenopause, production of these hormones slows down, but their effects on the body may continue. Androgens can lead to thinning hair, mid-abdominal fat deposits, and increased blood pressure and cholesterol levels.

The changes in the production of all hormones may wreak havoc in perimenopause by causing different symptoms and swings every day. Reading this book and figuring out how to stabilize the unstable is the first step to taking control of these midlife changes.

Hot Flashes Coming and Going (and Coming)

Hot flashes — also called hot flushes, or night sweats when they occur at night — are the most common symptom of menopause. The medical term for these events is *vasomotor symptoms* (VMS), and over 80 percent of women experience them at some point in menopause. About 50 percent of women experience these flashes during perimenopause, although they may not have VMS as frequently.

A *hot flash* can best be described as a sudden and intense feeling of warmth, especially in the upper body and the face. Increased perspiration often accompanies this feeling of warmth, and women who experience night sweats often remove blankets, sheets, and even their clothing to try to reduce their body heat. Sometimes, hot flashes are accompanied by a sensation of the heart racing, palpitations, and even dizziness or temporary shortness of breath.

Hot flashes are triggered by a drop in estrogen levels. Because perimenopause is a time of irregularly produced estrogen, your estrogen level may drop multiple times a day, triggering a hot flash each time. Women have often described these episodic flashes as a feeling that their internal thermostat isn't working properly. The drop in estrogen sends a signal to the brain to release adrenaline, causing a fight-or-flight reaction. Hot flashes aren't dangerous and are usually temporary, but a study conducted by Dr. Dongshan Zhu, Dr. Hsin-Fang Chung, and Dr. Gita D. Mishra, published in the *American Journal of Obstetrics and Gynecology* in 2020, suggests that women who have severe vasomotor symptoms may be at greater risk for future heart disease.

Hot flashes that occur in the middle of the night can cause interrupted sleep. Waking up perspiring and damp can make it hard to fall back asleep, and multiple nights of poor sleep can lead to more mood swings, irritability, and poor energy during the day.

If you're experiencing flashes that are causing a decrease in the quality of your sleep and your life, you have many ways to find relief, which I outline in Chapter 6.

Weathering Mental and Emotional Changes

Midlife can present you with plenty of new opportunities, and just as many challenges. Some of these challenges appear as new mental and emotional stressors. Just when you think you have a handle on dealing with family, work, responsibilities, and life events, perimenopause presents you with a ton of new symptoms to add to the mix, such as moodiness, fatigue, headaches, and weight gain.

It may be hard to separate which symptoms are a result of perimenopause and which may be from other health or medical conditions. The mental and emotional challenges that appear as a result of hormonal changes probably won't interfere with your day-to-day functioning. Symptoms of perimenopausal emotional changes typically fluctuate with changes in hormone levels and tend to be episodic.

Telling sadness from depression

Medical professionals consider occasional moodiness, sadness, or anxiety normal, but researchers have seen a link between fluctuating hormones and depression.

A decrease in estrogen levels may happen at about the same time that you start to feel depressed or anxious, but doctors don't consider estrogen supplementation to work as a treatment for depression or anxiety. Even though some sadness or moodiness may seem normal while you age and your life changes in ways that you may not have expected, true depression doesn't pass. Sad feelings that are associated with life changes or sad events are temporary; depression is not.

WARNING

If, during this time of perimenopause, you also experience changes in your appetite, sleep, and activity levels, or a feeling that activities that used to bring you pleasure are no longer pleasurable, please get evaluated for depression. Don't just write these feelings off as a symptom of perimenopause — and don't let your doctor do that, either.

Handling perimenopausal anxiety

Anxious feelings may start to rise with the fluctuating hormone levels of perimenopause. At the time of hot flashes, you may experience what feels like anxiety because low estrogen levels trigger the brain to release adrenaline, and your heart may race in response. True anxiety occurs more than just in response to a hot flash. *Anxiety* is intense, excessive, and persistent worry and fear about everyday situations. It may seem that anxiety is occurring at the same time as hormonal fluctuations, but always have any pervasive anxiety evaluated if that anxiety interferes with activities in your daily life.

Keeping Things Sexy Despite a Low Libido

Remember when you used to think about sex all the time? (Oh, was that not you?) *Low libido*, meaning a decrease in the feelings or thoughts related to sex and sexual activity, is one of the most common complaints of perimenopausal and menopausal women. Libido is a complex issue. For many women, so many things must be just right for them to feel like initiating a sexual encounter that it's a wonder they ever have a spontaneous sexual thought. Sex drive may naturally decline a bit over the years, especially if you're in a long-term relationship and somewhat comfortable in your sexual habits (or lack thereof).

Hormone decline rarely is the sole explanation for low libido — all menopausal women have low hormone levels unless they take supplemental hormones, and plenty of menopausal women think about and want to have sex. Low self-esteem and thoughts about your own body while you age may play a role in a lack of desire to initiate sex. Relationship issues, stress, lack of good sleep, anxiety and depression, changing family situations, busy schedules, and discomfort during sex may all factor into a lack of desire for sexual activity — or, at least, a lack of desire to initiate it.

Sometimes, you must address all these other issues to regain the ability to initiate, or to be responsive to, a sexual encounter. (See Chapter 7 for more on your perimenopausal sexual life.)

Getting Your Brain out of the Fog

Have you ever misplaced your car keys? Forgotten the name of a neighbor, even while in the middle of a conversation with them? How many times do things like this have to happen to you before you begin to wonder whether you have reason to be worried?

Brain fog, lack of concentration, and memory issues are quite common while people age, and especially when women approach menopause. Researchers believe that hormonal decline does have something to do with changes in brain function because a lack of estrogen seems to cause memory and concentration changes. Declining hormone levels, specifically estrogen and progesterone, can also result in poor quality sleep, which in turn can result in poorer concentration and cognition.

Of course, decreasing hormone levels aren't the only cause of cognitive decline. Vascular disease, such as the kind caused by high blood pressure or heart disease, can decrease the amount of blood that flows to the brain, which can also cause a decrease in concentration and cognitive function. Conditions such as depression, dehydration, anemia, and thyroid disease, as well as stress, can all result in brain fog and memory issues.

Have a discussion with your doctor to figure out whether problems that you have with concentration are due to fluctuations in hormone levels in perimenopause or are a sign of more serious cognitive issues. They may have some suggestions on how to decipher whether something other than the changes of perimenopause are causing your fuzzy thinking. You probably have options that you can try to help the fog to lift, so discuss your brain concerns at your medical visit. (See Chapter 6 for more about keeping your brain healthy.)

Chapter **3**

Special Circumstances That Can Impact Perimenopause

All women age and go through life transitions. So many signs and symptoms that you may experience while you age fall into the category of The Normal Perimenopausal Transition. Hopefully, this book can reassure you about just how expected and normal many of these symptoms are in midlife.

But what if you don't have the medical history of an average 40-something-year-old woman? What if you've experienced medical conditions, surgeries, or illnesses that change the way that your body experiences perimenopause and even menopause? What if you can't follow the normal playbook on how you'll feel and what to expect?

In this chapter, you can find out about some medical conditions, diagnoses, and surgeries that may affect how you go through your menopausal transition. Eventually, all women who reach a certain age experience menopause, and most women have some type of perimenopausal transition in the years prior. But specific life events may have you experiencing that transition, and the care that you receive, differently. If you fall into any of these categories, take a deeper dive into this chapter to get some information that may be specific to your individual journey.

Recognizing How Diverse Health Journeys Can Affect Perimenopause

Perimenopause, the transitional phase leading to menopause, isn't a one-size-fits all experience. It's a complex physical, hormonal, and cognitive adjustment. Not all women experience the same symptoms, and those symptoms don't occur to the same extent with every woman.

There are, however, certain special circumstances — relating to health history and genetics — that can significantly influence how you experience this transformative period. For instance, anything that changes your organs of reproduction (your uterus or ovaries) or changes the normal stimulation and release of hormones or hormonal signals can potentially change the course of your transition to menopause.

Medical conditions

The following section discusses some conditions that can impact what a woman experiences during this transition.

Polycystic ovarian syndrome (PCOS)

Polycystic ovarian syndrome (PCOS) is a condition that affects about 10 percent of women; usually, a medical provider diagnoses this syndrome in your 20s or 30s. This syndrome occurs when the ovaries produce an abnormal amount of male sex hormones, also called *androgens*. The ovaries normally produce androgens in small amounts, but if you have high levels of androgens in your body, your ovaries don't ovulate regularly, which causes some very common and specific symptoms:

» Disruption in the normal monthly menstrual cycle

» Periods that are longer or shorter than average, or that vary widely in interval from month to month

If you have PCOS, you may find it difficult to tell whether you're actually in peri-menopause because of the irregular menstrual cycles that you experienced all of your adult life. However, you may have more of a handle on how to deal with irregular periods than women who always had regular menstrual cycles prior to entering perimenopause.

You treat PCOS in very similar ways to how you treat perimenopause; your doctor and you can manage the symptoms of mood swings, poor sleep, fatigue, and irregular bleeding with the suggestions that I offer in Chapters 6, 9, and 13.

But with PCOS, there are other things to consider:

>> **Fertility:** If you want to become pregnant and have been diagnosed with polycystic ovarian syndrome, it's a good bet you'll need some reproductive assistance because your ovaries don't ovulate on a regular schedule.

>> **Uterine lining:** If you have no period-like bleeding for months at a time and aren't yet menopausal, your doctor will want to assess the lining of your uterus to make sure that in all those months without a period, you're not getting a thick build-up of blood and endometrial lining inside the uterus, which can result in precancer or cancer of the uterus.

Your doctor can check the lining of your uterus by using either an ultrasound machine or a small camera that goes inside the uterus (a *hysteroscope*).

Even if your menstrual patterns don't seem to change much, have a medical eval-uation when your periods start to skip more than five or six months because your PCOS symptoms may make it hard to tell whether you're going through a peri-menopausal transition.

Women who have PCOS may have different symptoms, depending on which type of PCOS they have. I outline the different types in the following sections.

Insulin-resistant PCOS

Insulin-resistant PCOS is the most common type. It occurs when your body stops responding appropriately to insulin and this causes the levels of sugar in your bloodstream to increase. This blood sugar increase triggers an increase in the production of male hormones, which keep ovulation from occurring regularly. Women who have this type of PCOS often have these symptoms:

>> Dark patches of skin in their skinfold areas (the neck, groin, and armpits)

>> Acne, especially on the jawline and in the skinfolds

>> Fatigue

>> Overweight or obesity

Insulin is a hormone that the *pancreas,* a gland in the abdomen, produces. The pancreas secretes insulin response to increased amounts of *glucose* (sugar) in the blood. Insulin helps transport glucose into your muscle, fat, and liver cells, where it's converted into glycogen or fat so that your body can store it for later use when your body needs energy. Worsening insulin resistance leads to Type 2 diabetes.

Inflammatory PCOS

Inflammatory PCOS occurs when your body suffers from chronic inflammation, which can interfere with ovulation and your menstrual cycle. The inflammation also drives up the production of male hormones (*androgens*). Sometimes, targeting the source of inflammation can help relieve the symptoms. Symptoms can include

>> Headaches

>> Joint pain

>> Fatigue

>> Skin issues, such as eczema

>> Bowel issues, such as inflammatory bowel syndrome

Post-pill PCOS

This temporary and uncommon condition may occur after you discontinue taking long-term hormonal birth control. Your body may experience a surge of *androgens* (male hormones) after you stop taking a birth control pill or using other hormonal contraception. The symptoms (weight gain, irregular periods, acne, and irregular hair growth on the body, face, or chest) typically go away in several months.

Adrenal PCOS

Your adrenal glands are two small triangle-shaped glands, one located on top of each of your kidneys. They produce hormones that help regulate your metabolism, immune system, blood pressure, stress response, and many other essential functions. One of the hormones that they produce in response to stress is DHEA (dehydroepiandrosterone).

When you are under lots of stress for a long period of time, your adrenals may produce elevated levels of DHEA, which can cause many of the same symptoms as other types of PCOS; irregular or missed periods, acne, weight gain, fatigue, and hair loss or growth.

Premature ovarian failure (POF)

Premature ovarian failure (POF), also called *premature menopause*, can occur at any age prior to the natural time that menopause should occur. At whatever age you receive this diagnosis, it means the end of natural fertility because it signals an end of ovarian function. So the ovaries no longer ovulate or produce hormones (estrogen, progesterone, and testosterone). Premature menopause occurs in about 1 in 100 women, and a variety of conditions can leave a woman susceptible to it:

>> Genetic disorders

>> Autoimmune disorders

>> Severe anorexia or other disordered eating

>> Nutritional deficits and severe weight loss or weight gain

>> Chronic, severe physical stress

>> Damage to the blood supply of the ovaries during other, unrelated surgery

>> Pituitary tumors

Because premature ovarian failure, and the symptoms that come along with it, occur so much earlier than menopause or even perimenopause would usually occur, the diagnosis may not even be on your or your doctor's radar.

REMEMBER

POF is rarely reversible. Sometimes, if you and your doctor catch it early enough and it's caused by a medication or treatable condition, your ovaries might restart and function again. But this reversal doesn't happen often. Your healthcare provider usually needs blood test results for the diagnosis, but your doctor has to think of that possibility in the first place, causing them to order those tests and get an answer.

History of endometrial ablation

Endometrial ablation is a procedure designed to destroy (*ablate*) the lining of the uterus with the goal of reducing or eliminating bleeding from menstrual periods. Your doctor can perform this procedure in a hospital operating room or in an office setting. They insert tools through the vagina and cervix into the uterus, and then use those tools to access and destroy the endometrial layer of your uterus.

Medical professionals can use several methods to achieve this ablation:

>> Cold

>> Heat

>> Electrosurgery

>> High-energy radio frequency

Doctors don't usually recommend this procedure in women who have certain uterine conditions, such as unusual anatomy. You also can't have a uterine ablation if you have cancer or an active pelvic infection, or if you may want a future pregnancy.

WARNING

Be aware that uterine ablation comes with some risks, such as pain and infection, as well as possibly damage to the surrounding bowel or bladder if the ablation touches an unintended area or makes a hole in the uterine wall (called a *perforation*).

If you had an endometrial ablation procedure that successfully diminished or eliminated your menstrual bleeding, congratulations! You likely don't have to endure one of the most annoying symptoms of perimenopause — irregular, heavy, or random bleeding.

An ablation doesn't affect your ovaries or the signals that come from your brain that trigger the ovaries to make certain hormones at certain times of your cycle, so the other aspects of your menstrual cycle aren't affected by this procedure.

REMEMBER

You may still have all the other perimenopausal symptoms when your ovaries start to slow down: brain fog, PMS, mood swings, poor sleep, vaginal dryness, weight gain, poor concentration, and irritability. You just don't have to worry about any irregular periods added to the mix. It may take a little more investigation or a little more experimentation to determine when and if you are in perimenopause, but if your age is right and the symptoms match up, your healthcare provider can help treat the symptoms you do have.

High risk of breast and/or ovarian cancer

If someone in your immediate family has (or has had) breast or ovarian cancer, your risk for these cancers goes up. If first-degree relatives have breast cancer (your mom, your sister, or your daughter), your risk of developing breast cancer is more than two times the risk of someone who has no family history.

You may want to take a test to see whether you carry a genetic mutation that increases your risk for breast and ovarian cancer. You can also research whether someone in your family carries these genes.

Medical science can currently screen for many mutations, including BRCA 1 and 2 (the letters BRCA stand for *BReast CAncer susceptibility gene*). Many other gene mutations besides BRCA 1 and 2 also exist. If you test for these genes and the results show that you do carry one of these mutations, your lifetime risk for developing breast and ovarian cancer increases greatly. You can reduce your risk through surgeries, medications, and surveillance plans if you do carry one of these genes.

But how does this cancer-risk knowledge affect your perimenopause? Scientists are still trying to work that out. Some studies suggest that carriers of the BRCA 1 and 2 gene mutation experience their natural menopause at an earlier age than the average age of 51.

Most medical societies believe that doctors can treat perimenopausal and menopausal women who carry these genetic mutations similarly to how they treat women who don't carry those mutations, as far as treatment for symptoms is concerned. Here are some points to keep in mind about treatments for those in this high-risk group:

>> **Treatments:** Women who carry genetic mutations should have access to all medical and hormonal treatments to relieve their perimenopause and menopause symptoms. This is a plan that they must make in shared decision-making with their medical provider.

>> **Hormone therapy:** You may feel hesitant to use menopausal hormone therapy if you know that you carry a mutation that increases your risk of developing cancer. Have a discussion of the individual risks and benefits of this therapy with your healthcare provider, making them familiar with your medical and family history.

>> **Surgery:** One of the recommended risk-reducing treatments for women who carry the BRCA 1 or 2 genetic mutations (among other mutations) involves removing the fallopian tubes and ovaries as soon as the woman no longer wants to have children. Some women may also choose to have a surgery to remove all of their breast tissue (bilateral mastectomy). This may seem like a drastic surgery to undergo, especially if you do not yet have a cancer diagnosis, but it is also a risk-reducing procedure to consider.

REMEMBER

Surgery substantially reduces the risk of breast or ovarian cancer in the future. Of course, removing ovaries prior to menopause results in surgical menopause, regardless of the age at which the surgery is performed. (See the sidebar "Surgically induced menopause," in this chapter, for more on surgical menopause.)

Procedures

The following sections describe procedures that, if you've undergone them prior to perimenopause, can affect your transition.

Hysterectomy

A *hysterectomy* is a surgical procedure where all or part of the uterus is removed. The term *hysterectomy* refers only to the uterus. Many women have the mistaken idea that it means also removing the ovaries. A surgeon can remove ovaries at the same time that they remove the uterus but depending on your age and the reason for the surgery, the surgeon often leaves the ovaries in place. If you have only your uterus removed, menstrual bleeding immediately ceases, and of course, you can't become pregnant in the future. If the surgeon doesn't remove your ovaries, and you're not yet in menopause, those ovaries should continue to function, making hormones and ovulating in the same way that they did prior to the hysterectomy.

Some studies suggest that women may go into menopause a little earlier after having a hysterectomy than they would if their uterus remained intact. But, in general, if you're under the age of 51 at the time of the surgery and your ovaries are still in place, those ovaries continue work until the typical age at which you would experience menopause naturally. As I discussed in the preceding section when talking about an endometrial ablation, when you go through your perimenopausal transition after a hysterectomy, you don't have the random or irregular periods that are a hallmark of midlife. However, you may have all the other perimenopausal symptoms (which I talk about in Chapter 2), and you can treat them however you and your medical team see fit.

RECOGNIZING MENOPAUSE IF YOU DON'T HAVE A UTERUS

A 54-year-old new patient was referred to my office via a friend. She had a *hysterectomy* (removal of the uterus) at age 45 for very heavy bleeding during her periods. She kept her ovaries. About a year after the surgery, she had a blood clot in her leg that traveled to her lungs (called a *pulmonary embolism*). Now, at age 54, she complained of poor concentration, irritability, and night sweats which caused her to have poor sleep.

She had some questions: How would she know when she was in menopause because she didn't have the signal of no periods for 12 months to tell her that she was there? Also, how could we relieve her symptoms?

Even though we couldn't rely on an absence of periods because she had no uterus, the combination of being 54 and having menopausal symptoms tells me all I need to know to diagnose her as menopausal. Her ovaries were likely not working any longer, and I could offer her some options when it came to relief. However, a patient who has had a blood clot, especially one that traveled to the lungs, can't utilize estrogen therapy, at least in oral form, because estrogen supplementation can increase the risk for blood clots. The medical community still hasn't agreed about whether she could safely use transdermal (through the skin) estrogen, but I chose to try some options from my list of alternatives to see whether I could help her find relief. She felt much better after trying a supplement to relieve her hot flashes.

Ovary removal

Your doctor may recommend removing your ovaries surgically for many different medical reasons. You may have

>> Suffered from large or recurrent ovarian cysts

>> A worrisome tumor on your ovary

>> A twisted ovary, cutting off its blood supply (also called a *torsion*)

>> A serious infection on your ovary

>> *Endometriosis* (a condition in which tissues of the uterus grow outside the uterus)

>> A hysterectomy when you were very close to menopause and had the ovaries electively removed

SURGICALLY INDUCED MENOPAUSE

Any time a woman has both ovaries removed before she has reached the age of menopause, she immediately enters what's called *surgical menopause* post-operatively. Surgical menopause is the most extreme and fastest entrance into menopause. When the surgery begins, the patient isn't in menopause. But when she wakes up in the recovery room, she is. Menopausal symptoms may begin immediately, including hot flashes and night sweats, that the patient wasn't experiencing prior to the surgery. If your healthcare provider recommends removing your ovaries, have a discussion prior to the surgery about managing immediate menopausal symptoms.

If your doctor determines it's safe to do so, start menopausal hormone replacement within a day or so of surgical recovery, to minimize the severity of menopausal symptoms. You and your healthcare team can then titrate the doses and type of

(continued)

(continued)

treatment over time to relieve symptoms of this quick and immediate transition to menopause. If your situation precludes hormone therapy, then talk with your doctor about some type of alternative treatment for symptoms that may present soon after the operation.

Following menopause-inducing surgery, you may experience any or all of the following symptoms, just like with naturally occurring menopause (which you can read about in Chapter 2):

- **Hot flashes:** You may experience hot flashes with varying frequency and at different times of day. These hot flashes sometimes occur at the same time as heart palpitations, and you can find them irritating and uncomfortable. The good news is that they may not last long.

- **Emotional shifts:** Like with any hormonal change, surgery that induces menopause can cause you to feel fluctuating emotions, including irritability, a drop in confidence, and a loss of concentration and memory.

- **Impact on sex life:** A common symptom of menopause involves vaginal dryness and discomfort, both of which can understandably deplete your sex drive or make sex painful.

Chemotherapy or radiation therapy

Women who have a cancer diagnosis often have a combination of treatments, including surgery, chemotherapy, and radiation therapy, depending on what type of cancer they have and where it's located in the body. These common cancer treatments may cause ovarian failure:

» **Chemotherapy:** Drug treatments that use powerful chemicals to kill fast-growing tumor cells in your body or prevent new cancer cells from growing

» **Radiation therapy:** A treatment that uses high doses of radiation to kill cancer cells and shrink tumors

These treatments may cause temporary or permanent cessation of ovarian function. This condition has a similar effect as having premature ovarian failure (see the preceding section), where all the symptoms of menopause start to occur much earlier than they would have naturally.

With ovarian failure due to cancer treatment, you likely don't experience a peri-menopausal transition nor a slow move toward menopause with gradual and worsening symptoms. Menopausal symptoms can all just start overnight. Again, have a discussion with your healthcare provider about the options for treating the probable symptoms and consequences of chemotherapy and radiation before you experience them.

REMEMBER

Many women who undergo cancer treatment (as well as their treating clinicians) focus so intensely on survival that they may not discuss the hot flashes, vaginal dryness, and extreme fatigue that may come along with premature chemo- or radiation-induced menopause. But having that conversation and having a plan can really help you improve the quality of your life post-cancer treatment.

A HYSTERECTOMY DOESN'T TRIGGER MENOPAUSE

A long-time patient started seeing me when she was 38 years old. At the time, she reported having had two vaginal deliveries and didn't plan on any further pregnancies. She was on a birth control pill and had regular monthly periods. Several years later, at age 43, while still on these pills, she started having very heavy and irregular periods. She also reported feeling very irritable and moody, so we switched to a different pill. Then she started bleeding in between her periods, so I had her get a pelvic ultrasound.

This ultrasound showed that she had several *fibroids* (benign growths) in her uterus and a very thick buildup of the lining inside the uterus — thicker that it should have been for someone on a birth control pill. I biopsied the lining, and it wasn't something dangerous, such as cancer.

After a long discussion, this patient decided that she wanted to have a hysterectomy, rather than to continue (for what might have been years) on contraception or other forms of medical management. She felt it was worth the surgery because, after a hysterectomy, her discomfort and bleeding problems would be gone. She had her hysterectomy (and maintained her ovaries), and at age 45, she feels comfortable — and, so far, no perimenopausal symptoms have appeared.

Chapter **4**

Examining Genetic and Environmental Influences

Because you're reading this book, you may want to be informed about your own perimenopausal transition and the symptoms you may be having. Or maybe you're interested because someone you love is going through this phase of life. You may think that everyone in midlife is feeling the same: "We're all tired, sleeping poorly, bleeding irregularly, and having mood swings." But *does* everybody feel the same? Why do some women seem to have minimal symptoms and others feel wildly unstable? Why do some women bleed like they're in the middle of a crime scene and others barely notice that their periods have slowly left the building?

Like almost everything else in life, your genetics and your environment are two factors working in consort to make you who you are. You may be able to control some factors to help make your midlife years more enjoyable, but you have absolutely no control over other factors. (You can't change your family history or your genetics — at least, not yet!)

In this chapter, you can find out how your individual history, your family's history, and your environment may play a role in the type of menopausal transition you experience. I look at how old patterns and habits may influence your current quality of life and whether you can do anything to combat what might seem to be your destiny.

Your Individual History: Sleuthing Out Clues

Although perimenopause may be affecting your memory (see Chapter 6 for more on perimenopause-related memory issues), we all have some very specific memories about dealing with our menstrual and reproductive history. You can gather clues from several places:

>> Your teenage years (or even earlier if your period started before you hit 13)

>> What your menstrual periods used to be like, in length of time that you bled, how heavy the monthly periods were, and how regularly you experienced your period

>> Any pregnancies

>> Your general medical health and wellness

Use this information as a roadmap for what to expect in perimenopause and beyond.

Looking at your menstrual and reproductive history

Although it may now seem like a very long time ago, most women have some type of a specific memory about their first menstrual period. You became aware of menstruation somehow:

>> The Talk with your mom or another female relative or friend

>> The class in middle school in which you had to watch a video about puberty

>> A pamphlet that someone handed you to read

>> A library book that someone checked out for you that provided an explanation of what menstruation is all about

And that very first menstrual period has something very ceremonial and memorable about it. Whether you look back on it with horror or happiness kind of depends on what kind of preparation you had.

Most girls begin to menstruate somewhere between the ages of 11 and 13, although it can start as early as 10 and as late as 15 and still be considered within the normal age range. But does the exact age at which you experienced that first period affect the age at which you'll see your last one? Does an early beginning lead to an early end, as far as reproductive life is concerned? Doctors agree that the timing of a woman's first period likely doesn't relate to the time that she begins menopause.

Many women believe that if they started menstruating at an early age, menopause will also occur at a younger age; they believe that menopause occurs when a woman runs out of eggs. But, women are born with millions of eggs, and most of those eggs are never used. The timing of menopause has more to do with the aging of the eggs and factors that may speed up the egg-aging process.

The results of some studies show a correlation between the age of a woman's first period and the age of menopause, and some study results don't. The medical community doesn't yet have a consensus on this potential connection. Whether there's a connection between the start of menstruation and the start of menopause, the age of the onset of menstruation in the United States has gotten slightly younger on average, but the average age of menopause hasn't changed: It's still 51, and most women go through menopause between age 47 and 56.

Thinking about the menstrual cycles of your younger years

Some lucky young women can always plan around their menstrual cycle. They start having periods around the expected time (such as age 13) and know exactly when their period will start every month; they can count 28 days forward — and boom, menstruation starts again. If they're very lucky, the period isn't too intrusive; lasting only three or four days, not too heavy, not too painful; and every month, like clockwork, they experience the same scenario. Who are these women? These are the women that are experiencing the normal, textbook menstrual cycle.

If the preceding paragraph describes you, you had a very lucky set of reproductive years because experiencing periods like this makes it easy to plan, easy to figure out when you're most likely ovulating, and easy to know when you're most likely starting to go through perimenopause. For you, lucky reader, perimenopause is obvious because your periods start to become irregular. You begin to experience irregularities and unusual bleeding patterns for the first time. Instead of 28 days in between your periods, there will be 30, 36, or 40 — or more or less. You can put a label on it — this irregularity signals your perimenopause.

But what about the rest of us? If you never had perfectly timed, regular intervals to your periods, you may struggle a little to figure out whether you've started perimenopause. If your periods have always and forever had no pattern, rhyme, or reason, seeming to come at random intervals, perimenopause may be happening before you even realize it.

If you're used to skipping your menstruation some months, followed by random or surprise periods, you may need to pay attention to some of the other perimenopausal clues to decide whether you're making a transition.

One interesting study, published in the journal *Menopause* in 2022, concluded that women who have shorter menstrual cycles, defined as less than 25 days in between, are more likely to reach menopause earlier than women who have average-length cycles (26 to 34 days).

Reflecting on your pregnancies

During pregnancy, the natural process of ovulation is temporarily stopped. Do pregnancies somehow delay the process of the ovaries aging, leading to a later onset of natural menopause? Possibly. Many studies tried to answer that question, but no studies had enough participants to draw any conclusions until a Norwegian study in 2021, which included over 30,000 women.

The researchers concluded, in an article published in the *Journal of Human Reproduction* in 2022, that women who had no childbirths entered menopause at the earliest ages, and those who had three childbirths had menopause at the latest ages. Although the study collected the data by using questionnaires (which are sometimes problematic because the women filling out the questionnaires may not remember clearly), because the number of participants was so high, the investigators felt comfortable drawing reasonable conclusions.

Factoring in PMS

You may experience the delightful symptoms of premenstrual syndrome (PMS), or even premenstrual dysphoric disorder (PMDD), including depression, anxiety, and mood changes. PMS and PMDD refer to a group of symptoms that typically occur between the middle of the menstrual cycle (ovulation time) and the onset of the next period.

Doctors don't understand this syndrome very well, but it likely involves the hormonal changes that occur throughout the menstrual cycle — especially the changes that occur in the weeks before you begin your monthly period. Symptoms may include mood swings, tender breasts, food cravings, irritability, depression, bloating, and brain fog. Sound familiar? Yes — you *can* have perimenopausal symptoms and PMS at the same time! (Yay.) Because PMS and perimenopause share many of the same symptoms, you may have difficulty figuring out whether your symptoms are related to PMS or to perimenopause.

Keeping a calendar or a diary that has all your symptoms and when they occur in relation to periods may help to clarify:

>> **Consistent:** If this combination of symptoms seems to occur only in the days or weeks leading up to the onset of your period, disappear after the bleeding begins, and then recur the following month on the same schedule, you likely have PMS symptoms.

>> **Inconsistent:** If your symptoms seem to appear randomly throughout the month and are paired with typical menopausal symptoms, either in between or simultaneously (hot flashes, night sweats, insomnia, vaginal dryness, low energy), you're experiencing PMS at the very same time that you're transitioning to menopause, so you have both sets of symptoms simultaneously (and I'm so sorry).

TIP

If you think you may be experiencing PMS and perimenopause symptoms at the same time — good times! — you have a very good reason to seek treatment. (See Chapter 10, where I talk about how physical and emotional changes are caused by the hormonal swings of perimenopause.)

Understanding endometriosis and fibroids

Endometriosis and fibroids are two common disorders that are associated with estrogen:

>> **Endometriosis:** A disorder in which the tissue that normally lines the inside cavity of the uterus grows abnormally, outside the uterus. This tissue, called *endometrial tissue,* can be found on the ovaries, fallopian tubes, or intestines. Estrogen can stimulate the tissue, so when estrogen is present, the tissue can grow, causing symptoms of pain, cramps, headaches, irregular bleeding, and heavy periods. See Figure 4-1 for an illustration of where endometrial tissue can grow.

>> **Fibroids:** Non-cancerous growths that develop in various areas of the uterus. They can grow anywhere inside or outside of the uterine body and can be as small as a raisin or as big as a basketball. Estrogen can stimulate fibroids, also called *myomas,* to grow, potentially causing symptoms such as pain, cramps, pressure, and heavy or prolonged periods. Figure 4-2 shows an illustration of where fibroids may form.

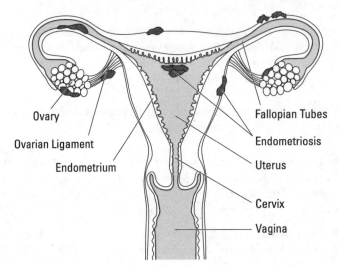

FIGURE 4-1:
A pelvic cavity with areas that can develop endometriosis highlighted.

Ovary

Ovarian Ligament

Endometrium

Fallopian Tubes

Endometriosis

Uterus

Cervix

Vagina

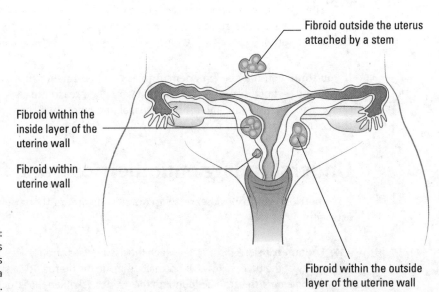

FIGURE 4-2:
Various sizes and positions of fibroids in a uterus.

Fibroid outside the uterus attached by a stem

Fibroid within the inside layer of the uterine wall

Fibroid within uterine wall

Fibroid within the outside layer of the uterine wall

By the time you reach perimenopause, you likely already know whether you have fibroids or endometriosis. Again, symptoms tend to be worse during periods because of the presence of hormones, especially estrogen, which can have a stimulating effect on both conditions. In perimenopause, the level of estrogen rises and falls unevenly, so endometriosis and fibroids may worsen and cause more symptoms during this time.

WARNING

If you have had a long history of heavy, painful, or irregular bleeding and think that you may have one of these conditions, perimenopause is *not* the time to just wait it out. Get an evaluation by a medical professional — because, during perimenopause, hormone levels swing widely, so symptoms are likely to worsen. Doctors can offer many treatments that can help relieve worsening symptoms over a potentially years–long perimenopausal transition.

Asking Your Loved Ones About Their Menopausal Transition

Even if you never had that early talk with your mom or your female relatives about what their first period was like, talk to them now about their experience of menopause. Genetics and family history play a strong role in determining a woman's age at menopause and how exactly she'll experience her own menopausal transition.

Keep these facts in mind when discussing your family members' experiences:

>> The age of menopause is defined as one year after the final menstrual period and is on average about 51 years old. The years leading up to this menopausal state are considered perimenopause.

>> Some women naturally enter menopause much earlier than average, and some much later.

>> Menopause can occur because of certain conditions, such as medical illnesses, chemotherapy, very high or very low body mass index, and certain medications.

>> The age of natural menopause is most influenced by family history. If your mother experienced her natural menopause early, then you probably will, too.

You can also predict your age at menopause if you have information about multiple relatives, such as sisters, aunts, and grandmothers. If most of the women in your family, including your mother, experienced their menopause at similar times — whether early, late, or somewhere in between — you can plan for the approximate time of your menopause with some confidence.

REMEMBER

Because the age at which family members entered menopause is only one factor that can influence the timing of your own perimenopause and menopausal transition, if you don't have that history, you're still not really unprepared. Reading books such as this one and becoming well informed on what changes you're likely to experience will help you to have a healthy midlife experience and help you to anticipate the many physical and emotional changes that will come your way (if they haven't already).

Reviewing Your Personal Habits and Medical History

Although doctors haven't yet proven a 100 percent certain cause and effect, some aspects of your medical history and your health habits very likely influence how and when you go through your perimenopausal transition. The following sections go into just a few personal habits and pieces of medical history that can influence when you'll probably begin your transition to menopause, as well as what symptoms you'll experience — and to what extent you'll experience them.

Smoking

The onset of perimenopause occurs one to two years earlier in women who smoke than in women who don't smoke. Smoking seems to have an impact on the speed with which the ovaries age, and it also may affect the speed with which estrogen is made in or removed from the body. In perimenopause, hormone levels are already swinging from high to low. Consider trying to quit now if you're a smoker.

Medications

Any medication that can damage your ovaries or affects the ability of your ovaries to make estrogen can cause hormonal changes that lead to perimenopause and, eventually, menopause. Chemotherapy drugs used in certain cancer treatments can slow down or turn off your ovarian function. Depending on the type of chemotherapy, these ovarian changes may be temporary, or they may be permanent.

Certain medications that are designed to affect the ovaries, such as medications to treat endometriosis or fibroids, can cause a medically induced perimenopause or menopause. Depending on your age when you start these medications, the effect on the ovaries can be temporary or permanent.

Hormonal contraception, by design, can stop ovarian function, thus halting ovulation to prevent pregnancy. You may want to take hormonal contraception (or continue taking it) during perimenopause if you don't want to become pregnant. (Chapter 10 talks more about birth control during perimenopause.)

You can find a lot of misinformation about the possible long-term effects of hormonal contraception (the birth control pill, patch, vaginal ring, injection, and the under-the-skin implant) out there. All of these forms of contraception prevent pregnancy by stopping ovulation while you have that contraceptive in your system. Except for the injectable contraceptive (a shot every 12 weeks), all the others have no long-term effect on ovarian function after you stop using them.

But if you start a birth control pill at age 35, take it continuously for five years, and then stop taking it, you *will* be less fertile after going off it. The decrease in fertility doesn't have anything to do with the pill — it's because you're now 40 years old, and fertility naturally declines as you age. The birth control pill didn't have any type of long-term effect on your ovaries.

Medical conditions

If you've had an auto-immune disease your whole adult life (rheumatoid arthritis, lupus, thyroiditis, scleroderma, or other connective tissue diseases), you may expect to hit perimenopause and, eventually, menopause at earlier than the average age. These diseases affect the immune system, which normally protects your body from illness and invaders, making it go into overdrive and start attacking your own body's cells. The cells under attack can include those of the ovaries, and estrogen production can slow or stop at an early age because the ovarian cells that produce estrogen have been damaged.

Women who have seizure disorders may also have a risk of earlier transition to menopause both from the medications to treat the disease and from the effect of seizures on the brain's signals. Diabetes — especially Type 1, or Type 2 that you don't have under good control — can cause an earlier menopausal transition because the ovaries stop working sooner in response to higher sugar levels in the bloodstream.

Alcohol intake

Women who have a high alcohol intake may have earlier perimenopausal transitions for a couple of reasons:

>> **Liver damage:** Alcohol may affect the functioning of the liver, where some hormones are made and metabolized.

The liver produces binding globulins that assist the hormones estrogen and progesterone, along with thyroid hormones and cortisol, throughout the body. Damage to the liver impairs its capacity to metabolize and inactivate estrogen.

>> **Poor nutrition:** Sometimes, increased alcohol leads to poor nutrition and vitamin deficiencies, slowing ovarian function and estrogen production.

Alcohol also seems to exacerbate the symptoms of perimenopause, increasing hot flashes, night sweats, and insomnia.

Extreme weight fluctuation

As far as perimenopausal timing and symptoms go, weight is one topic where you probably want to fall in the average range, which is a body mass index (BMI) of 18.5 to 24.9:

>> **Too little body fat (a BMI under 18.5):** Women who are very thin, have very little body fat, or have eating disorders such as anorexia or bulimia often have ovaries that don't function normally. Being too thin affects an area of the brain called the hypothalamus, which causes signals to the ovaries to diminish or shut down. This decrease in signaling may be temporary and reversible, but studies do link women who have eating disorders to earlier menopause.

>> **Too much body fat (a BMI over 24.9):** Having excess body fat, being overweight or obese, also influences your experience in menopause and perimenopause. One of the most important concerns most women have when they enter midlife is the fear of weight gain. Having excess body weight prior to the menopausal transition can make gaining more weight around the time of the menopausal transition more likely. Lower estrogen levels trigger a redistribution of body fat and a likelihood to gain more weight around the middle.

Carrying excess belly fat also increases health risks for heart disease, diabetes, and vascular disease.

WARNING

Surgeries

A *hysterectomy* is an operation where surgeons remove the uterus. Women have hysterectomies for various reasons, including pain, heavy bleeding, fibroids, cancers, or precancerous conditions. If you have your uterus removed prior to going through your menopausal transition, you may wonder how you'll know whether you're in perimenopause, or even in menopause. It depends. If you still have your ovaries and they're still functioning, don't assume that you're in menopause just because you have no more bleeding. (Remember — no more uterus means no more menstrual bleeding because the uterus is the source of that bleeding.)

At some point, those ovaries slow down and then cease to function. At that time, you'll probably experience the typical menopausal symptoms: hot flashes, night sweats, insomnia, mood swings, and so on. If you're experiencing those symptoms, you don't need an investigation with blood tests or imaging to know that you're in menopause.

Figuring out perimenopause may be a bit harder after a hysterectomy because you don't have irregular bleeding to clue you in, but if your other symptoms occur randomly or periodically, and you experience mood swings and irritability, you're probably in the perimenopausal transition phase.

If you had surgery where your ovaries were removed (called *oophorectomy*), you don't need blood tests or further investigation: You *are* in menopause. Removing ovaries renders you completely without your estrogen factory. No estrogen production = surgical menopause. Having your ovaries removed usually means sudden onset of menopausal symptoms, except in one instance: If you were menopausal prior to the surgery, removing the ovaries doesn't make much difference because they were already not functioning.

If you weren't in menopause prior to the surgery and start menopause immediately afterward, be prepared for a sudden drop in estrogen, which may lead to severe menopausal symptoms, such as hot flashes and night sweats. Please, please prepare for these changes by talking to your doctor about the many ways to ease that transition.

Exercise habits

A regular fitness routine can provide you with so many benefits while you go through your menopausal transition. Exercise and regular physical activity have a ton of benefits for all aspects of your health and life, and if you've never gotten into the habit of regularly moving your body, symptoms at this stage of your life can provide you motivation.

Exercise offers a ton of benefits for anyone:

>> Improves your ability to cope with stress

>> Helps with mood swings

>> Improves sleep

>> Keeps your heart healthy and your cholesterol low

>> Decreases the risk of many chronic conditions, including diabetes, high blood pressure, and osteoporosis

This is just a sampling of the benefits — the complete list goes on and on.

TIP

If you haven't decided to make regular exercise a part of your routine, do it now. Even moderate exercise, such as walking 30 minutes five times a week, has health benefits for your body and your mind. Regular exercise can also decrease the severity of perimenopausal and menopausal symptoms, increase your flexibility, and decrease your chances of experiencing a bone fracture.

2
Hormone Fluctuations and Their Impact in Perimenopause

IN THIS PART . . .

Adjust to changes in your menstrual cycle.

Understand the hormonal shifts of perimenopause.

Navigate sexuality and changes to your libido.

Chapter 5

Bleeding Is Such a Bother: Too Little, Too Much, Too Random

O ne of the first signs that you probably noticed about being over 40 was that you couldn't count on your period anymore. Maybe you never could count on it. Or maybe you knew when to expect your period by the symptoms that you'd start to have before the menstrual bleeding started. Maybe your period came like clockwork. Whatever pattern you got used to in your 20s and 30s, after you reach this time of midlife, you probably notice that things have changed. After age 35, and certainly after 40, the body tends to go through some changes that result in disruptions to your menstrual cycle.

In this chapter, you can explore what exactly happens to the parts of your reproductive system that are responsible for menstruation. Brain signals need to make their way to the ovaries, ovarian hormones need to talk to your uterus, and you have numerous feedback loops throughout to let the brain know how all these body parts are reacting to all that signaling.

Dealing with Menstrual Irregularity

At midlife, you may start to skip your period for a month or two when that never happened before. You may have heavier bleeding for more days than you're used to. Or maybe you find yourself buying large pads or super tampons when you haven't needed those for many years. After you pass age 35, you probably start to experience menstrual irregularities, and many things can influence what type of irregularities you have.

Of course, some lucky women have no changes in their period and sail through the perimenopausal years barely noticing a difference. Those women probably don't read a book such as this one, looking for answers. I also don't often see them in my medical practice.

Maybe you're not sure whether you ever did have normal menstrual periods. By definition, a menstrual period interval (the time from the start of one period to the start of the next one) can be anywhere from 23 to 35 days and still be considered normal. If you got your period exactly every 28 days or every 30 days on the dot, the medical community considers that not only normal but also *regular*.

What begins to happen during perimenopause is the onset of *irregular* cycles. There are many different types of irregularities (discussed in the following section) and many different reasons for them (which you can read about in the section "Identifying the Causes of Menstrual Bleeding Patterns," later in this chapter).

Evaluating Bleeding Patterns

As a young teenager, you probably had The Talk with your mom, a sister, or a close friend or relative who told you a bit of information about what to expect when you got that inevitable first period. Maybe it was a short conversation, but it probably included breaking the news that you would go through this cycle for many years to come and that while you bleed, you have to make use of some type of a sanitary product (now called feminine hygiene products or personal care products).

When you reach the age of perimenopause, sadly, no one makes it their business to have another, similar conversation. No one (often not even your doctor or a trusted medical professional) tells you that you'll once again experience menstrual periods that may plague you and disrupt your life, and that you may need to get reacquainted with various feminine hygiene products that you haven't had to look at for years. If you know what to expect, this transition may get a little easier, like The Talk may have made getting your first period easier.

During midlife, you might experience any number of changes in your menstrual cycle. The following sections give you some facts and information about possible changes to your period during perimenopause.

Skipped periods

Skipped periods occur when a month or more goes by with no sign of menstrual bleeding. In your younger days, you may have had periods that came every month, and you knew exactly when each one would arrive. So, it may come as a big surprise when that next expected period just doesn't appear. If you're a sexually active woman who has male partners, you may first think that you might be pregnant. (Whether this thought occurs with a sense of panic or one of hope depends, of course, on your situation. But many home pregnancy tests get used for just such an event.)

I see many midlife women in my gynecology practice who come in for a visit because of a skipped period. When I inevitably suggest we first do a pregnancy test, most of these women are skeptical. "I'm sure it's not that," they say. I ask, "Are you sexually active?" To which they answer, "Yes, but I'm over 40, so it's not pregnancy." I'm not sure why they dismiss that possibility, but I always check. At least five times in the past 10 years the test was positive, and the patient was shocked.

If your periods in your younger days have always been irregular, then a skipped period in your 40s may not raise any eyebrows (or any concerns). Your periods may just continue to follow a pattern that has been your normal, irregular period pattern. If you're familiar with this pattern, you already had it evaluated by your physician, and it doesn't disrupt your life (and as long as you know you aren't pregnant), you may continue with this normal pattern when you enter perimenopause.

More frequent periods

When your period comes more frequently than once a month, especially more frequently than every 23 days, medical professionals consider that an abnormally short menstrual interval. Your periods may have started out coming monthly, and then slowly through your midlife years, they snuck into an every-26- or every-24-day pattern over time. It's normal for period intervals to shorten while you age. However, such frequent bleeding can affect your quality of life if it goes on for too long. If that's the case, ask your doctor about the possibility of lengthening the interval with medications or evaluating possible reasons for these changes.

Heavier periods

It may happen suddenly, or it may happen gradually, but you may notice that your periods get heavier while you get older. You may notice heavy clots, bright red bleeding, and menstrual cramps that you haven't experienced for at least the last several years.

"What the heck is going on?" you may wonder while these heavy, clotty periods now become your dreaded norm. A heavy menstrual flow can affect your health and your quality of life, causing exhaustion, headaches, and dizziness. If you've always had heavy menstrual periods, you may not notice such a big change; but don't ignore periods that get suddenly heavier in midlife. See your healthcare provider so you can figure out if the heavier bleeding is just one of those perimenopausal adjustments your body is making, or if further evaluation or treatment is warranted.

Lighter periods

It sounds like a dream: progressively lighter periods while you go through your 40s, until they just fade away altogether at the appropriate time, never becoming bothersome, inconvenient, or symptomatic. For some women, that's exactly how they experience their perimenopausal menstrual changes. Sadly, the majority of women don't.

If you notice this pattern with your menstruation, you generally don't have a reason to worry, and you don't need to rush out for a medical evaluation. But you may want to mention the change to your medical provider at your next midlife check-up visit.

Longer periods

The average length of bleeding time per period is about 3 to 7 days. You may find that during this perimenopausal time, the number of days you bleed seems much longer; 9 or even 12 days of bleeding. Typically, these longer periods follow this pattern:

>> The first few days look like your normal menstrual-bleeding pattern.

>> The following few days see heavier bleeding.

>> Your period ends with about a week of bleeding that trails off, seeming to go on and on, but with only a little bit of bleeding or spotting each day.

This pattern creates a feeling that you're bleeding throughout the month, without much of a break. Sometimes, the bleeding lasts for a few days and then stops, only to return after a day or two of no bleeding. This additional bleeding doesn't reflect the start of a new period; it's the left-over bleeding from the period that just finished. Either of these patterns probably interferes with your quality of life, so talk to your doctor periods that suddenly seem never-ending.

Surprise periods

You may have gotten accustomed to your regular (or irregular) bleeding pattern. You can use a period tracker or a calendar to map out when you expect your next period to start. You plan around this knowledge and anticipate the days you need to wear certain clothes or buy certain products because of anticipated bleeding. You feel comfortable that you're navigating this time of midlife menstrual instability successfully — and then it happens. You're on a beach vacation, two weeks before you expect your next period to start, but here it is. Unexpected bleeding.

REMEMBER

Most incidents of surprise periods aren't dramatic or life-altering, but periods showing up at unexpected times are a hallmark of perimenopause — so like a Boy Scout, always be prepared.

No periods

Eventually, your periods will just go away. The average age of menopause is 51 years old. The definition of *menopause* is 12 consecutive months with no period. Of course, you can only own this title after the fact; after 12 months have passed. Until those 12 months have passed, you may go through a few episodes of almost-menopause, when you have no period for 3 months (or even 11 months), and then your period returns. So, you're not yet in menopause. The longer that you go without bleeding, however, the more likely that you're approaching menopause.

WARNING

Any bleeding that occurs after 12 menstruation-free months have passed doesn't mean that your period has returned. Bleeding again after the 12 period-free months is called *post-menopausal bleeding,* which can signal cancer, so have yourself evaluated by a healthcare provider.

Bleeding patterns that require immediate attention

WARNING

Although almost all bleeding patterns in perimenopause signal the normal hormonal changes of this transitional period, a few bleeding patterns should throw red flags. If you experience any of these bleeding patterns, make an urgent appointment with your doctor:

>> **Post-menopausal bleeding:** If you make it all the way through the 12-month no-period transition and therefore are in menopause, then suddenly you start having vaginal bleeding, visit your healthcare provider. This *post-menopausal bleeding* may not be a sign of something worrisome, but you need to rule out conditions such as cancer.

>> **Heavy sudden bleeding:** If you start to consistently have heavy, clotty, painful periods that last longer than your previous periods, and/or are noticeably heavier than your previous periods, have your situation evaluated by a medical professional. Heavy sudden bleeding can be a sign that you have something new like a tumor or a polyp growing inside your uterus. And heavy bleeding for months can cause anemia and other medical problems.

>> **Additional debilitating symptoms:** If your menstrual bleeding is accompanied by increasing abdominal or lower back pain, headaches, dizziness, nausea, or vomiting, have yourself assessed in a doctor's office.

Identifying the Causes of Perimenopausal Bleeding Patterns

To understand why menstrual bleeding patterns can change, first consider how they generally work in your reproductive years.

A normal uterus, which is a muscular organ, measures about 3 to 4 inches from top to bottom and 2 inches wide at its widest part. The uterus contains three segments:

>> **Fundus:** The broadest part of the uterus, at the top, where the fallopian tubes connect to the uterus

>> **Body:** The part of the uterus directly below the fundus that continues downward until the uterine walls and cavity begin to narrow

>> **Cervix:** The lowest region of the uterus that attaches to the vagina

The uterus also has three tissue layers, all of which you can see in Figure 5-1:

>> **Serosa:** The outermost layer

>> **Myometrium:** The middle, muscular layer

>> **Endometrium:** The inner lining of the uterus. This is the layer that sheds during menstruation

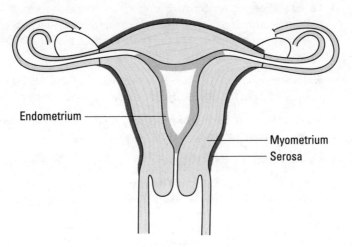

Endometrium

Myometrium
Serosa

FIGURE 5-1:
Anatomy of
a uterus.

Female reproductive organs are more than just the uterus, though:

>> **Ovaries:** The reproductive organs located near the fallopian tubes (which connect to the uterus) in which eggs are stored and certain hormones are produced

>> **Fallopian tubes:** Ducts that can transport an egg from an ovary to the uterus

>> **Vagina:** The canal from the cervix that leads outside the body

During the menstrual cycle, the uterine lining (the *endometrium*) gets thicker and rich with blood (which is the blood that sheds during menstrual bleeding).

Anatomical changes

Anatomical factors can affect your menstrual cycle. These are physical changes that occur within the reproductive system which can occur at any time. You may have anatomical changes to the structure of your uterus, cervix, and ovaries, as well as changes to how those structures function.

The anatomical changes that can occur in the uterus and cause irregular bleeding patterns include fibroids, polyps, pre-cancer or cancerous cells, and endometriosis (all shown in Figure 5-2):

>> **Cancerous cells:** These may be found in any part of the reproductive system, and cause irregular or unusual bleeding. Cancerous cells on the cervix, in the vagina or in the uterus are usually responsible for unexpected or irregular bleeding patterns.

>> **Cervical changes:** Abnormal cells may grow on the cervix that can be pre-cancerous, cancer, or benign (non-cancerous). Any atypical or abnormal cells that appear on the cervix can cause irregular bleeding, especially (but not always) at the time of sexual activity.

>> **Endometriosis:** A condition in which tissue similar to the lining of the uterus grows outside of the uterus. This is usually accompanied by pelvic pain.

>> **Fibroids:** Noncancerous growths of the uterine muscle that often appear during childbearing years.

>> **Ovarian cysts:** Fluid-filled sacs that can form on the ovaries.

>> **Polyps:** These are growths that develop on the inner lining of the uterus (the endometrium). They are usually non-cancerous but can contain cancer cells.

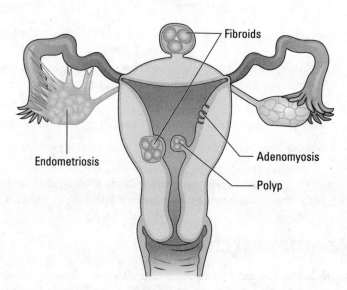

FIGURE 5-2:
Potential uterine abnormalities.

Irregular ovulation

The ovaries produce most of the hormones needed to prepare the body for reproduction, a process that follows these steps:

1. The brain (specifically the pituitary gland) produces follicle stimulating hormone (FSH) in the first few days of menstrual bleeding.

2. The FSH stimulates the ovary to produce estrogen (mostly estradiol).

3. In response to the production of estradiol, the uterine lining (the endometrium) builds up a thick lining of blood and tissue in preparation for the implantation of a fertilized egg.

4. The brain then produces luteinizing hormone (LH), which triggers the ovary to ovulate (release an egg).

5. After ovulation, a cyst forms from the left-over ovulation. This is called a corpus luteum cyst, and it produces progesterone to further prepare the uterine lining for an implanted embryo.

6. If there is no pregnancy, the corpus luteum disintegrates and progesterone and estrogen levels decrease.

7. The menstrual period begins again, and the entire cycle repeats itself.

While you get older, and certainly while you approach menopause, ovulation slows down or becomes irregular. (For this reason, fertility takes a deep dive after age 35, and especially after age 40.) If you don't ovulate, the corpus luteum in your ovaries doesn't produce progesterone.

If the ovaries don't produce progesterone in the regular monthly cycle, the lining of the uterus doesn't know when to shed. It may

>> Still shed on time, resulting in continued normal-interval menstrual cycles

>> Shed later than usual, resulting in delayed menstrual cycles

>> Not shed at all, adding layers to the endometrium each time the brain tells the ovaries to release estrogen, until the lining becomes so thick that it results in a heavier, longer period

Simply stated, during perimenopause, you ovulate irregularly, which causes many of the irregular bleeding patterns you may see.

Hormonal

The hormonal changes that occur during perimenopause usually cause the irregular bleeding patterns that you may see. Hormonal factors play a significant role in regulating the menstrual cycle, and therefore when those factors change, your cycle also changes. While you age, the production of hormones such as estrogen and progesterone becomes inconsistent and eventually declines, which deregulates your menstrual cycle. This hormonal decline can lead to changes in the timing, duration, and flow of menstrual bleeding.

A combination of factors

Of course, anatomical and hormonal changes can occur simultaneously, and each can exacerbate the others' impact. For example, hormonal irregularities can contribute to the development of anatomical abnormalities such as fibroids, and vice versa.

Correcting Various Bleeding Patterns

Of course, you and your doctor need to figure out the likely cause of your irregular bleeding before you can decide on the best course of action to correct it, or even if you need to correct it. The treatments you can consider depend on the cause of the bleeding pattern.

Anatomical treatments

If, after evaluation by a medical professional, you determine that you have an anatomical reason for your perimenopausal bleeding pattern, you likely need an anatomical solution. Doctors may be able to remove fibroids and polyps, biopsy your *endometrium* (the inner lining of your uterus) to check for cancer, and evaluate and treat pre-cancerous conditions. Cancer of the uterus or cervix is usually treated surgically (usually with removal of the uterus, also known as a *hysterectomy*).

Hormonal treatments

If you determine that hormonal changes are most likely causing your irregular or bothersome bleeding pattern, you need a hormonal solution. In perimenopause, you have available many and varied safe hormonal solutions to correct, lessen, or eliminate unwanted or bothersome bleeding. Your healthcare provider and you can consider hormonal contraception, hormone replacement, hormone blockers, and hormone modulators, depending on your individual situation, history, and safety profile. (See Chapter 6 for more on hormonal changes.)

IN THIS CHAPTER

» Understanding the menstrual cycle

» Riding the hormone rollercoaster

» Looking at birth control options in perimenopause

» Considering hormonal treatment options

» Treating perimenopause changes with non-hormonal options

Chapter **6**

Hormonal Changes: Understanding the Swings of Perimenopause

O ne of the major functions of sex hormones involves preparing the body to produce life. You probably have some type of memory of a middle school lecture or a pamphlet that tried to explain the connection between your impending need for monthly menstrual protection and the eggs that your ovaries were about to start releasing.

During perimenopause, you may sometimes feel like you're revisiting that time in your life: where you need someone to explain to you what's happening to your body. And for good reason: To understand what's happening hormonally in perimenopause, think back to the changes that you experienced when you entered puberty; think of how you felt at that time and how confusing it was for your body to be changing.

In this chapter, you can gain an understanding of what exactly happens with your hormones in perimenopause and why it all makes you feel so crazy and out of sorts sometimes. The wild swings in hormone levels at this time in your life can cause physical and emotional changes that make you feel like puberty is happening all over again.

So, what exactly do you do about all these hormonal changes in perimenopause? What can you do? Not to worry; there are many possible ways to reduce the effects of hormonal shifts at this stage, which you can read about in this chapter.

Understanding How Hormones Work During Your Reproductive Years

Hormones are responsible for most of the changes that occur in a woman's body while they enter their reproductive years, also called puberty. The physical changes, the mood shifts, the realization of sexual feelings all start to happen around the same time, usually around age 13. So how much do you truly understand about how hormones work in your body?

You may go about your daily life, experiencing the ebbs and flows of your menstrual cycles without giving it a second thought. But behind those monthly cycles lie a complex set of hormones and hormonal interactions. The following sections look at how your hormones change and shift, both during your early monthly cycles and while you age.

Going through the average monthly cycle

The average menstrual cycle interval is 28 days — meaning there are approximately 28 days from the start of one menstrual cycle until the start of the next one.

Figure 6-1 illustrates the hormones of a normal menstrual cycle.

During the bleeding phase of the menstrual cycle, the body (the uterus) is flushing out its lining because no embryo (an early pregnancy) was implanted in the uterine wall.

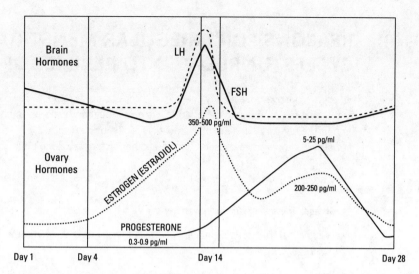

FIGURE 6-1:
Hormone levels
throughout the
menstrual cycle.

Here are the hormones at play throughout the menstrual cycle:

>> **Estrogen:** Produced in abundance in the ovaries from the time of puberty until the age of perimenopause. Estrogen plays a major role in many physical and mental systems in the body (energy, restful sleep, upbeat moods, sharp memory, strong bones, and a healthy heart, to name a few), not just in the reproductive system. Estrogen stimulated the lining inside the uterus to build up.

>> **Progesterone:** After you ovulate, your estrogen levels reduce slightly, and another hormone is released: progesterone. Progesterone is produced in the ovary, in the left-over remnants of the ovulated egg, and peaks at about day 21 of the cycle. Progesterone stabilizes the lining of the uterus and prepares it for a pregnancy.

>> If the egg that your ovary released is fertilized, the progesterone level stays high. But if the egg isn't fertilized (so no pregnancy), the estrogen and progesterone levels drop, and soon after, menstruation occurs again (Day 28, or what would also be Day 1 of the next menstrual cycle).

When all the hormones discussed in the preceding list are working in cyclical concert, you experience a predictable pattern of bleeding, moods, and physical and emotional changes that occur at predictable times during the cycle. Many women say that they know when they're ovulating, and some experience specific and predictable physical and emotional symptoms in the days and weeks leading up to their next menstrual period.

REASONS FOR IRREGULAR MENSTRUAL CYCLES (UNRELATED TO PERIMENOPAUSE)

Of course, not everyone's body keeps to the perfect, predictable 28-day cycle described in this chapter. Although in this chapter, we cover the many ways perimenopause can impact the regularity and other characteristics of your menstrual cycle, irregular menstrual cycles can also be caused by various other factors and conditions.

Here are some common reasons that your period can be less than regular:

- **Stress:** Physical or emotional stress can cause changes in your menstrual cycle.
- **Weight fluctuations:** Significant changes in body weight, whether weight gain or weight loss.
- **Exercise intensity:** Extreme or sudden increases in exercise, as well as intense training routines.
- **Thyroid disorders:** Conditions such as hypothyroidism or hyperthyroidism.
- **Contraceptive use or change:** Starting or stopping hormonal contraceptives or changing the type of contraception.
- **Uterine fibroids or polyps:** Noncancerous growths in the uterus (called *fibroids*) or small, benign growths on the uterine lining (called *polyps*).
- **Endometriosis:** A condition in which tissue similar to the lining of the uterus grows outside of the uterus.

  Adenomyosis: A condition similar to endometriosis, but where the lining of the uterus grows into the muscle layer of the uterus.
- **Pelvic inflammatory disease (PID):** Often caused by untreated sexually transmitted infections.
- **Breastfeeding:** The hormonal changes associated with breastfeeding.

  These hormonal changes can also cause *amenorrhea* (complete absence of menstruation).
- **Certain medications:** Some medications, such as certain antidepressants or antipsychotics.
- **Substance abuse:** Excessive use of alcohol or drugs.
- **Travel or time zone changes:** Rapid shifts in time zones that temporarily affect the body's internal clock.

Changes to your menstrual cycle while you age

Around your mid-30s, some of the hormone signals that you can read about in the preceding section may start to malfunction. This breakdown may happen because of age alone, medical conditions, certain medications, or a combination of these factors.

In relation to your age, hormones shift because of changes happening in your ovaries. During perimenopause, sometimes you ovulate and sometimes you don't. Here are the hormone culprits behind irregular periods in perimenopause:

>> **Inconsistent follicle-stimulating hormone (FSH):** Sometimes, the brain produces enough FSH to get the ovaries to do their job and produce enough estrogen. If your cycle goes as expected, you continue to have the energy, restful sleep, and emotional stability that estrogen provides.

 Sometimes your brain doesn't produce enough FSH, and sometimes your ovaries just don't respond to it. When either of these events happens, you get estrogen produced in spurts and starts, sometimes up and down in the same day.

>> **Ineffective luteinizing hormone (LH):** Right at the time you're supposed to be ovulating, you may have a weak LH surge, or your ovaries just don't respond to it. Therefore, the ovaries may produce some varying amounts of progesterone, or none at all. And so your next period may be on time, late, or nonexistent. This variation in the effectiveness of LH leads to the irregularity of menstrual cycles that are the hallmark of perimenopause.

So, in short, the menstrual cycle is all messed up! Estrogen levels go up or down in response to stimulation from the brain, but often not in any regular, predictable way:

>> **Low estrogen levels:** When your estrogen levels go down, you experience the symptoms most associated with menopause: hot flashes, night sweats, low energy, vaginal dryness, low libido, and brain fog.

>> **Normal estrogen levels:** When your estrogen levels go back up, the low-estrogen symptoms temporarily vanish, and a menstrual period will return — but bleeding may occur at irregular intervals or be heavier than normal.

 Normal estrogen levels without progesterone: When ovulation and, consequently, progesterone are missing, you may experience symptoms of premenstrual syndrome (PMS), including emotional instability, fatigue, acne, brain fog, slower digestion, and bloating.

Fluctuating Hormones and Missed Periods: The Possibility of Pregnancy

When you enter perimenopause and experience the hormonal shifts that come with it, you must consider the possibility of pregnancy. I've encountered in my practice numerous patients who believed, because they were experiencing symptoms of perimenopause, that they couldn't become pregnant.

In fact, not only can you become pregnant — even when you're skipping periods — it should be considered as a possibility.

>> **Women at 40:** At age 40, the chance of a spontaneous pregnancy is approximately 5 to 10 percent. Chances of pregnancy decline every year after that, but women can potentially get pregnant at any time that they are still having menstrual periods, even if they are rare or irregular.

>> **Women over 50:** Although unintentional pregnancies become increasingly rare for women over 50, statistics show that a very small number of women who engage in unprotected sexual intercourse at age 50 may still become pregnant.

Sometimes, a missed period is a result of the hormonal miscommunication discussed in the preceding section: missed signals and temporary ovarian dysfunction. In these cases, if you continue to wait, after an extended period of time, the next menstrual period will likely appear.

However, don't get caught in this scenario during perimenopause: Months have passed, no period in sight, and you're experiencing the symptoms that match up with perimenopause in full force — fatigue, poor sleep, changes in appetite.

You finally make a visit to the doctor to help manage these symptoms — and unexpectedly, the pregnancy test is positive. Although you may find pregnancy at age 45 a happy surprise, an unplanned pregnancy may not be something you want or are prepared for at this age.

Considering the Benefits of Birth Control

After your menstrual periods become irregular, you always need to consider the possibility of a pregnancy, even if only to plan how to avoid it. You can choose from many forms of hormonal contraception that will help avoid an undesired pregnancy, while at the same time stabilizing or eliminating the heavy and irregular menstrual bleeding that comes along with perimenopause.

ORAL CONTRACEPTION: THE PILL

Years ago, the medical community thought that older women of reproductive age shouldn't use hormonal contraception, especially a birth control pill. Doctors worried that women in their later 30s or 40s could be more at risk for complications such as blood clots, high blood pressure, or heart conditions.

However, a more recent medical perspective on contraception, including birth control pills, shows that certain, specific doses and hormone combinations can work effectively and safely for women in midlife who need both contraception and cycle control. Both the American College of Obstetrics and Gynecologists and the North American Menopause Society recommend that women may continue contraceptive use up until age 50 to 55 if there are no medical contraindications (such as uncontrolled high blood pressure or vascular disease).

Talk with your doctor about which of the methods of birth control discussed in the following sections may work best for you in your individual situation.

REMEMBER

If you need some form of birth control, and you also want some way to get a handle on irregular bleeding, emotions, and other symptoms caused by the unstable hormones in perimenopause, explore which method may best take care of both at the same time.

Combination pills

Birth control pills are mostly combinations of the hormones estrogen and progesterone. Different pills have different strengths of estrogen and different chemical formulas of progesterone/progestin. Most birth control pills provide a stable dose of these two hormones daily, taking over for ovaries that have started to produce fluctuating amounts of estrogen and progesterone in perimenopause.

TECHNICAL STUFF

Combination birth control pills prevent the ovaries from releasing an egg; and if an ovary still somehow releases an egg, the pill also slows the egg's progress through the fallopian tubes and thickens the mucous at the cervix, both of which make fertilization of that egg more difficult.

Birth control pills have two major benefits:

>> **Pregnancy prevention:** When taken correctly, oral contraceptives are over 98 percent effective in preventing pregnancy.

>> **Hormone regulation:** By delivering stable amounts of hormones daily, birth control pills can regulate the menstrual cycle; and there are some specific pills that are known to help with mood swings and emotional instability that may occur at any time, but especially in perimenopause.

Combination birth control pills can have side effects, and not all women are candidates to take them. They can cause

>> Breast tenderness

>> Headaches

>> Nausea

>> Bloating

>> Acne

>> Increased blood pressure

>> Breakthrough bleeding (bleeding in between periods)

The most serious potential side effects of birth control pills, although very rare, include

>> Blood clots in the legs or lungs

>> Gallbladder disease

>> Stroke

>> Liver cancer

Women who have a history of liver disease, migraine headaches that include an aura, uncontrolled high blood pressure, blood clots, or certain cancers can't take combination birth control pills because of the increased risk of these serious side effects.

Combination birth control pills come in different mixtures of *active* (hormone-containing) and *placebo* (inactive) pills, depending on when and how often you want to have your periods:

>> **Conventional dosing:** These packs usually contain 21 active pills and 7 inactive pills. Some have 24 active and 4 inactive pills. Bleeding likely occurs monthly on the days you take the inactive pills.

>> **Extended-cycle dosing:** You take an active pill for 84 days, then 7 days of placebo pills. Bleeding generally occurs only four times a year, during the time that you take the inactive pills.

>> **Continuous dosing:** Some birth control pill formulations contain only active pills that you take continuously, which eliminates bleeding altogether.

Doctors also categorize combination birth control pills based on whether the dose of hormones in the active pills stays the same throughout the pack or the doses vary.

>> **Monophasic:** Every active pill contains the same amount of estrogen and progesterone.

>> **Multiphasic:** The amount of estrogen and progesterone vary based on which week of the pack you are in.

Progesterone-only pills

Some birth control pills contain only progesterone and are called (kind of obviously) progesterone-only pills (POPs). In each pack of pills, all the pills contain the same amount of the hormone progesterone or *progestin* (a synthetic form of progesterone), and the pack contains no inactive or placebo pills.

Women who can't or don't want to take estrogen typically use these progesterone pills. (also sometimes called the *mini-pill*):

>> Slows an egg's progress through the fallopian tubes

>> Causes the lining inside the uterus (the *endometrium*) to thin

>> Sometimes also suppresses ovulation, although not as consistently as a combination pill

It may or may not eliminate periods and provide cycle control, but it generally decreases the amount of bleeding per period.

Other forms of hormonal birth control

Several other hormonal birth control methods utilize a combination of estrogen and progesterone, in addition to daily pills:

>> **Birth control patch:** A contraceptive patch applied to the skin, usually on the lower abdomen or the arm, and changed weekly, with the last of four weeks considered patch-free. During the week that you don't wear a patch, having no patch (and therefore no hormones that the patch delivers) stimulates a menstrual period.

Healthcare professionals don't consider perimenopausal women ideal candidates for use of a combination patch because of possibly higher estrogen blood levels, (compared with oral contraceptives) which potentially can increase the risk for blood clots, but for some otherwise healthy women, it is a viable option.

>> **Vaginal ring:** This contraception uses a combination of estrogen and progesterone/progestin. It's a small, soft plastic ring placed in the vagina by a woman who chooses to use it and left in place for 21 days. You can then remove it and leave it out for seven days, during which the decrease in hormones stimulates a menstrual period. After 7 days, a new ring is inserted, again to be left in place for 21 days. This pattern is continued monthly. The hormones in the ring stop ovulation by using a very low dose combination of estrogen and progesterone.

Both the patch and the ring have the same side effect profile as a birth control pill, which I talk about in the section "Oral contraception: The Pill," earlier in this chapter, and they have a similar list of the reasons that you may not be a candidate.

Long-term reversible contraception

All hormonal contraceptives labeled *long-acting and reversible contraception* (known as LARCs) utilize progesterone in various formulas and doses. A doctor inserts the contraceptive device into your body, and that method can provide contraception for three to seven years. After inserted, these contraceptives provide excellent protection against pregnancy because their effectiveness doesn't rely on your ability to use or take them properly. Here are the leading LARCs:

>> **Intrauterine devices (IUDs):** Placed in the uterus by a doctor in an office procedure. An IUD lasts from three to seven years, depending on which specific IUD your doctor and you agree to place. IUDs don't stop ovulation, but they work at the level of the uterus, thickening cervical mucous and making it harder for a fertilized egg to make it into the uterus to implant there.

REMEMBER

>> **Hormonal IUDs:** Also called progesterone releasing IUDs, these devices usually change the regularity and amount of bleeding that occurs with monthly menstrual periods. Some women have no bleeding at all, some have spotting, some have irregular bleeding, and some have regular light periods. You can't know what bleeding pattern you'll have until after you have the IUD in place for several months.

>> **Subdermal implant:** A rod of progesterone (a different type than that used in hormonal IUDs) inserted into the upper arm, just under the skin. You usually

have this implant placed in an office procedure. It lasts up to three years and also changes the menstrual bleeding pattern in an unknown way. Some women have no bleeding at all, and the rest have any number of bleeding patterns from light and regular, to moderate and irregular, and anything in between.

>> **Progesterone injections:** An every-12-week shot of progesterone that suppresses ovulation and thickens cervical mucous.

All progesterone LARCs may have various side effects, including

>> Headaches

>> Depression

>> Skin changes, such as oily skin or acne

>> Appetite changes, including an increase or a decrease in appetite

>> Weight gain—if you have an increase in appetite, you may also see weight gain

>> Increased facial and/or body hair

USING BIRTH CONTROL FOR NON-CONTRACEPTIVE REASONS

Why does anyone use contraception if they're not at risk of getting pregnant? Maybe you had a permanent method of birth control performed, such as a *tubal ligation* (sometimes called "getting your tubes tied," but no actual tying goes on — this procedure simply blocks eggs from your ovaries reaching your uterus). Or maybe you're not sexually active, or your sexual partner is female.

Hormonal contraception provides many other benefits besides the not-getting-pregnant benefit. Pills, patches, rings, and LARCs all influence the amount and frequency of menstrual bleeding; if your doctor hasn't suggested a hormonal contraceptive as a possible solution for your perimenopausal bleeding and mood swings, ask them why they haven't! Of course, your healthcare provider and you need to take a thorough look at your history, your medical problems, your other medications, and your age before deciding whether this treatment is right for you.

(continued)

(continued)

Not every contraceptive is safe or appropriate for every perimenopausal woman. But your doctor and you can often find a good match because the very problems plaguing you in perimenopause are some of the exact things that various forms of hormonal contraception can treat effectively.

If the first pill that you try doesn't help your irregular bleeding, try a different strength, brand, or dose. Try an IUD or try a vaginal ring.

Perimenopause is a temporary period of time that may last up to seven years, and one of these methods may be just the bridge that you need until all the ovulations cease, all the bleeding stops, the emotional ride stabilizes, and you're firmly in menopause. (Yay?)

Treating Perimenopause Symptoms with Hormones

Hormone therapies to treat perimenopausal and menopausal women fall into two categories:

>> **Menopausal hormone therapy (MHT):** Prescribing a hormone or hormones — usually estrogen, progestin/progesterone, and sometimes testosterone — to treat the symptoms of perimenopause and menopause and to help keep your bones strong. Your doctor may prescribe MHT during your perimenopause to treat various symptoms and control irregular bleeding.

>> **Hormone replacement therapy (HRT):** The prescriptions replace hormones that the person doesn't naturally have anymore. Replacement doses are usually needed in special cases, where a woman has had premature menopause, or primary ovarian insufficiency.

Many women visit their doctor with complaints of perimenopausal symptoms, and their doctor tells them that they can't use hormone therapy (aside from contraceptives) because they're not in menopause. Does that position make any sense? If you don't have some other hormone or a particular vitamin in your body and that absence makes you feel miserable, the obvious solution involves simply replacing the missing ingredient in a dose that relieves those symptoms.

In the case of perimenopause, the missing hormone or hormones are usually progesterone, estrogen, testosterone, or some combination of the three.

Focusing on progesterone

Progesterone is produced by the after-effects of ovulation. Regular ovulation is the missing piece in perimenopause, so when women have poor sleep, emotional instability, irritability, and irregular periods, they're probably missing the production of adequate progesterone that normally comes from monthly ovulation. Taking progesterone can help relieve these symptoms and may be the only component of hormone therapy that you need.

Your doctor can prescribe progesterone-only hormone therapy in various doses and various formulations, and if one does not work, you can try a different dose, brand, formulation, or plan to see whether it is better at relieving your symptoms Any form of progesterone may have side effects, including

>> Breast pain

>> Mood changes

>> Headaches

>> Heartburn

>> Bloating or swelling

>> Hot flashes

REMEMBER

Progestins are the synthetic form of the natural progesterone that's made by the ovaries.

Here are some forms of often-prescribed progesterone that you may receive as treatment during perimenopause:

>> **Micronized progesterone:** A prescription of oral medication available under various brand names. It comes in doses of 100 milligram (mg) and 200 mg capsules. Manufacturers use peanut oil when making these pills, so you can't use them if you have an allergy to peanuts. The base material used to make these pills comes from plant sources, and the medication is chemically similar to the progesterone made in the ovaries.

>> **Progestin-contraception pills:** Also called the *mini-pill,* the most common type of *progestin* (synthetic progesterone) used is called norethindrone. Most progestin-only oral contraceptives contain 35 micrograms (µg) of norethindrone per pill and come in a pack of 28 identical pills.

LOOKING AHEAD TO THE CLARITY — YES, CLARITY! — OF MENOPAUSE

Navigating the perimenopausal phase can feel like a complex puzzle of hormonal ebbs and flows. However, while you transition into menopause, you have a silver lining awaiting you: clarity and simplicity. When you enter menopause, the rollercoaster of hormonal fluctuations levels out. For this reason, finding relief becomes far more straightforward. Instead of meticulously deciphering which hormone is causing what effect on a particular day, you face a far more stable hormonal landscape.

Administering the right dose of hormones to achieve relief becomes a streamlined process. It's a welcome shift from the perimenopausal maze, offering a sense of ease and predictability. Embracing menopause signifies a new chapter, free from the intricate hormonal dance — a time of steady equilibrium and the opportunity to truly savor the relief you've earned.

One newer progestin-only contraceptive contains a progestin called drospirenone in a 24/4 pill pack with 4 mg of drospirenone taken for 24 days and *placebo* (inactive) pills for 4 days. For some women, these drospirenone pills cause fewer of the side effects, such as bloating and headaches, that norethindrone can cause but drospirenone may result in other side effects, such as nausea, headaches, or mood changes.

» **Norethindrone acetate:** You usually take this progestin a in 5 mg or 10 mg oral tablet per dose. It works by increasing the levels of progesterone in your body. It can help regulate irregular bleeding and relieve some perimenopausal and menopausal symptoms.

» **Medroxyprogesterone acetate:** This oral progestin usually comes in doses of 5 mg to 10 mg orally daily. It can bring on a period that is late and treat perimenopausal irregular bleeding.

Hormone therapies

Your healthcare provider and you can choose from many ways to take progesterone or progestins to relieve the symptoms of perimenopause.

Cyclic progesterone

If you still have regular menstrual cycles, but your symptoms occur mostly in the week to ten days leading up to your next period, you may need to take progesterone or a progestin only in those ten or so days to get relief.

To put this plan in action, you need a calendar and knowledge of the date of your next expected period. The medical community calls it *cyclic use* because you take the progesterone or progestin only in the part of your menstrual cycle where symptoms occur.

Daily progesterone

If you experience symptoms of irritability, mood instability, poor sleep, and low energy throughout the month, regardless of bleeding patterns, sometimes taking progesterone daily can alleviate these symptoms. This regimen may

>> Relieve emotional perimenopausal symptoms

>> Lessen episodes of heavy menstrual bleeding

REMEMBER

Daily progesterone may sometimes result in increased irregularity in the menstrual cycle, but you may see the trade-off as worth it (better sleep and mood stability.)

Cyclic estrogen and progesterone

If your perimenopausal symptoms include hot flashes, low energy, night sweats, poor sleep, vaginal dryness, and aches and pains, you may need more than just progesterone for relief. These symptoms often respond to taking some estrogen, as well.

TECHNICAL
STUFF

However, if you're still having periods, your body is already making some estrogen. So why add more? Estrogen levels are swinging widely (and wildly) in perimenopause. Just like a traditional birth control pill attempts to create stability by using daily doses of estrogen and progesterone, a cyclic hormone regimen does the same, with much lower doses of estrogen than birth control pills contain. (Flip back to the section "Oral contraception: The Pill," earlier in this chapter, for a discussion of birth control pill options.)

If you take estrogen in the doses used for hormone therapy, you take it daily for most of the month (typically, 25 days), along with a daily dose of progesterone. You stop taking both hormones for the last five days of your cycle to allow any blood that has built up in the lining of the uterus (the *endometrium*) to shed.

Hopefully, this regimen addresses symptoms that you find bothersome through-out the month, and allows for controlled, expected bleeding episodes during the last few days of the cycle.

WARNING

This method is the most controversial and the most labor intensive because it involves not only taking estrogen (while your body is still making some estrogen), but also counting the days and taking estrogen on certain days of the month and progesterone or a progestin on others.

Menopausal hormone therapy

Estrogen plays such a large role in so many of your body's functions that compen-sating for the decreased production levels that perimenopause and menopause bring factors in as a key component of most hormone therapies.

Taking estrogen to relieve symptoms works very well, but it can cause other side effects, most notably building up a too-thick lining inside the uterus (in the *endo-metrium*). Therefore, if you haven't had your uterus removed surgically (a *hyster-ectomy*) and plan to start an estrogen therapy regimen, progesterone or a progestin in some shape or form should be added in to that plan to provide protection for the uterine lining by limiting the amount of blood and tissue that will build there. *Combination therapy* refers to a combination of estrogen and progesterone/progestin:

>> **Estrogen:** You can find estrogen available in pills, patches, creams, gels, and sprays — all designed to relieve hot flashes, night sweats, and other symp-toms that are caused by declining estrogen levels. The Menopause Society recommends estrogen that gets absorbed through the skin (*transdermal* estrogen) because it doesn't seem to increase the risk of blood clots, high blood pressure, or stroke the way that an estrogen taken orally, in a pill, can.

>> **Progesterone and progestins:** Available in pills, patches (as part of a combination regimen with estrogen) and vaginal formulations. By far the most studied form of progesterone is the pill that you take orally. If you had a hysterectomy, you may not need to take progesterone because the main function of progesterone in a hormonal program is to protect the endome-trium. Taking oral progesterone may also help with sleep and moods.

REMEMBER

Testosterone is a hormone also made in the ovaries, and some studies suggest it's connected to libido, because women taking testosterone sometimes report an increase in their sexual thoughts and desires. Some women may add testosterone into their menopausal hormone programs, but it's not FDA-approved for women nor available commercially for this purpose in the United States.

Daily estrogen and progesterone use

Menopause means everything is pretty much gone (hormonally speaking), so figuring out what dose of hormones you must take to get relief is infinitely easier than figuring out which hormone on which day is swinging in which direction.

Sometimes, a menopausal hormone therapy regimen works during perimenopause, as well — although not in all situations. Small doses of daily estrogen and progesterone on every day of the cycle may stabilize moods and bleeding patterns for those perimenopausal women no longer make much estrogen of their own but don't have episodes of heavy and irregular bleeding.

Heavy bleeding usually means that ovaries are still producing adequate amounts of their own estrogen in perimenopause, so adding more often results in even heavier and *more* irregular bleeding. But, in certain women and with certain doses, you potentially can use a daily combination regimen of estrogen with some type of progesterone/progestin to relieve symptoms and irregular bleeding.

Other combination regimens

To treat hot flashes, night sweats and many other menopausal symptoms we need to choose estrogen doses that are high enough to relieve those symptoms.

These doses may cause a thick lining of blood to build up inside the uterine cavity if you take them alone. A great way to make sure that you don't have this problem involves placing a progesterone-releasing intrauterine device (IUD) inside the uterus. The progesterone in the IUD will work to prevent the thick build-up of blood and tissue inside the uterus, and it can remain in place for years. (You can read more about IUDs in the section "Long-term reversible contraception," earlier in this chapter.) This combination can take you all the way through your perimenopausal transition and into menopause, providing relief of symptoms, as well as safety, with very little that you must think about.

Alternatives to Hormone Therapy

Some women can't participate in hormone therapy regimens for a variety of reasons:

>> **Medical reasons:** Some women can't use or take hormones because of medical conditions or a medical history that makes taking those hormones dangerous, such as breast cancer, liver disease, or a blood-clotting disorder.

>> **Personal reasons:** Some women just don't want to take any hormones for their own reasons, such as anxiety or a fear of taking hormones, or a family history that worries them. Prescribing hormones for perimenopausal and menopausal relief of symptoms is a decision shared by you and your doctor, so if you would prefer an alternatives, find someone who has some to offer you.

Luckily, some alternative therapies can help relieve the symptoms of perimenopause. You may be able to find one or a combination of products that can help relieve various perimenopausal or menopausal symptoms. Unfortunately, no single alternative product has evidence that shows it can relieve all of your symptoms.

TIP

Chapter 20 includes stories about perimenopausal management plans, some of which don't involve any hormone therapy.

Supplements

Generally, no government body regulates supplements — what they contain or what they claim to do — and some supplements can cause serious health problems. Try to stick with supplements that your doctor recommends and that have studies with evidence of safety.

WARNING

Don't take *black cohosh* to try to relieve your perimenopausal symptoms. This supplement mimics estrogen, which can relieve symptoms, but it also has the potential to cause heavier periods, and a build-up of the lining inside the uterus, with an increased risk of developing pre-cancerous cells (*hyperplasia*) and endometrial cancer (cancer of the lining of the uterus) in the same way that taking estrogen without progesterone can.

Supplements with evidence of effectiveness and safety

Although not many studies have been conducted, these supplements don't appear dangerous and may help your perimenopause symptoms.

WARNING

Of course, you may have an allergic reaction or experience side effects with any supplement, and the supplement might interact with medications you're taking, so always check with your healthcare provider before starting a supplement.

Here are the generally accepted non-hormonal supplements for hot flash relief:

>> **Equelle:** The recommended dose is one tablet in the morning and one tablet in the evening. This supplement uses *S-equol,* a compound made during the

fermentation of soy (so you can't take it if you're allergic to soy). It's a metabolite of soy *isoflavones* (meaning it has a similar structure to estrogen) and contains some calcium. Take it at least four hours before or after you take any thyroid medication.

>> **Estrovera:** A supplement that uses a compound called ERr 731, which is extracted from the root of a rhubarb plant. You take one tablet daily, with water and food, to decrease the incidence of hot flashes, irritability, and nighttime sweating.

>> **Relizen:** A tablet that contains Swedish flower pollen extract, which you take daily. The recommended dose is two tablets a day to provide relief from hot flashes and night sweats. Pollen extracts from a certain family of grasses are thought to relieve hot flashes, irritability, and sleeplessness. The exact mechanism of action is unclear.

>> **Tempo:** Contains a formulation of *genistein,* the primary isoflavone found in soy, so it can help to minimize menopausal symptoms. The dose is one tablet daily, and they're dissolvable, so you don't need a glass of water to take them.

Supplements that lack evidence of effectiveness

No significant evidence suggests that these supplements can alleviate your hot flashes and night sweats, although they each has anecdotal evidence that they can help:

>> **Ginseng:** A few studies have found some evidence that different types of ginseng may help improve your quality of life during menopause. It can potentially help with moods and sleep; however, no evidence suggests that it helps with the physical symptoms of perimenopause or menopause.

>> **Red clover:** Many women use red clover, hoping that its natural plant estrogens can help relieve some of their menopausal symptoms. No studies definitively prove that it can help safely relieve symptoms.

>> **Wild yam:** Pills and creams made from certain species of wild yam are popular alternatives to hormone therapy for menopause, but no research has shown that they work to treat menopausal symptoms at all.

Prescription medications

Some nonhormonal prescription medications may help relieve hot flashes. But only one nonhormonal medication is FDA approved for the treatment of hot flashes (fezolinetant). The FDA has approved all the other prescription medications in this list for other indications, but they may treat hot flashes as a side effect:

- **Amitriptyline:** A tricyclic antidepressant used also to treat insomnia, nerve pain, fibromyalgia, and headaches. Although doctors don't yet understand the mechanism of action through which amitriptyline relieves hot flashes and night sweats, it may increase levels of estrogen in the body as a side effect of treatment for other conditions. Taking this medication comes with several common side effects, such as nausea, dry mouth, and drowsiness.

- **Clonidine (brand name Catapres):** This blood pressure medication has a side effect of decreasing hot flashes in some women. If you have high blood pressure and hot flashes, this medication may be for you! It comes in a tablet or a weekly patch. You usually start at a low dose and then gradually increase it weekly until you reach a dose that relieves your hot flashes.

- **Fezolinetant (brand name Veozah):** Approved to treat hot flashes by the FDA in May 2023, this medication targets neurons in the brain that control temperature regulation.

TECHNICAL STUFF

These particular neurons are sensitive to estrogen, so when estrogen declines during perimenopause and menopause, the neurons get extra stimulation, which causes hot flashes and nighttime sweats. This drug works by blocking a receptor in the brain and therefore decreasing the firing of these neurons. The studies that led to the drug's approval showed that it reduced the frequency of hot flashes by about 60 percent.

This once-a-day pill is approved for women who have moderate to severe hot flashes up to age 65. Women who have liver disease can't take fezolinetant because it can cause the liver to function less efficiently and raise the levels of liver enzymes in the blood.

- **Paroxetine (brand names Paxil and Brisdelle):** Paroxetine falls into the category selective serotonin reuptake inhibitors (SSRIs), a type of antidepressant and anti-anxiety medication. It raises the level of a neurotransmitter called *serotonin* in your body, which may influence your body's thermoregulation, thus potentially decreasing hot flashes.

- **Topiramate (brand name Topamax):** Helps relieve migraine headaches and acts also as an anti-seizure medicine. Some small studies have shown it to effectively treat hot flashes and sweating in perimenopause and menopause. It comes in an oral capsule that you swallow, or one that you can open and sprinkle on soft food.

>> **Venlafaxine (brand name Effexor):** This anti-anxiety/antidepressant medication falls into the class of medication known as serotonin-norepinephrine reuptake inhibitors (SNRIs). It raises the levels of the neurotransmitter's serotonin and norepinephrine in your brain, which can incidentally influence your body's ability to regulate your body temperature.

HAVING A TREATMENT BACKUP PLAN OR TWO

While you try to make decisions about contraception, hormone therapy, and alternative treatments, ask your physician to review with you a list of risks and benefits. Discuss with them what will most likely work for you, given your individual history, symptoms, and circumstances.

And always have a backup plan in place. When you go through that list of options with your doctor, identify several approaches that might work. Always have something else as a possibility if the first (or second or third) choice doesn't help with your symptoms or has unpleasant side effects. Getting relief in perimenopause is a work in progress, and getting it right may be as close as the next item on your list.

Chapter **7**

Holding onto Your Libido and Keeping It Comfortable "Down There"

J ust like all other aspects of getting older, different people experience different changes in their desire for sexual activity, their degree of pleasure, and interest in being or remaining sexually active. Those changes depend on your history, your relationships, your past and current attitudes about sex and sexuality, and the physical and emotional changes that you may be going through.

REMEMBER

Don't believe the bill of goods that society tries to sell you — that having less sex and being less interested in sex while you get older is natural and normal. It's not. And don't think that women after a certain age can't be sexy or sexual. Dismiss those old-fashioned myths.

If you notice changes in your sexual relationship around midlife, you're not alone. These changes can happen for many reasons — and you have many ways to maintain or revive the sex life that you want. Thinking back on your relationship history and sexual desire history can give you a good marker to measure whether your sexual interest is noticeably changing at midlife.

If you've never been interested in sex or sexual physical relationships, never experienced sexual feelings or desires, and never truly felt sexually attracted to anyone, then after age 40, you probably won't have these feelings suddenly start to develop.

However, if you're noticing a significant change in your interest in sex and sexual activity when you pass age 40, and if this change is distressing to you or detrimental to your relationship, take a good look at some of the possible reasons for this change. You may be able to figure out some steps to take that can help return you to a time when you felt more interested in sex and sexual activities.

In this chapter, you can look at the physical, emotional, and hormonal changes that may affect your thoughts and attitudes, and cause symptom that can be extremely uncomfortable and limiting in terms of sexual activity.

What Is Libido Anyway, and How Does It Work?

Low libido happens for a variety of reasons, and a true and thorough investigation can help uncover both some of the causes and some of the possible solutions. Although a thorough investigation into loss of libido is beyond the scope of this book, this section includes some basic questions and information to help point you in the right direction.

Libido, as a term, describes sexual appetite or sex drive. Hormones, medical conditions, brain function, culture, relationship issues, learned activities, and past experiences all influence libido. Regardless of gender or gender identity, the same neural, hormonal, and chemical pathways in the body shape a person's sex drive and sexual appetite. These pathways can, in turn, stimulate sexual arousal and cause physical changes that we associate with sexual interest: flushing, sweating, engorgement or swelling in the genital area, and lubrication.

A set definition of a "normal" libido doesn't exist. Either a high or a low libido becomes a problem only if it interferes with relationships, sexual function, your well-being, or the quality of your life.

REMEMBER

Sexual attraction is only one type of attraction. People who are *asexual* (meaning they have no sexual feelings and aren't sexually attracted to anyone) may still identify as straight, gay, bisexual, or queer. Love doesn't have to equal sex, and you can have strong meaningful relationships with partners that don't necessarily involve sex. If you've felt uninterested in sex your whole life, the changes in perimenopause probably won't cause major changes in your desires.

If you've always had a low sex drive, have never really been interested in sexual encounters and relationships, and you don't find that fact distressing, you probably won't have a problem in midlife when you find that your interest stays about the same.

But if spontaneous sexual interest was effortless and important to you in your younger years, having to work on it a bit while you age doesn't mean you aren't sexy, interesting, or fun. Feeling that old spark may be just a bit more complicated and take a little more time.

Many factors can potentially cause low libido. If you're feeling a difference in your sexual interest, investigating whether the cause falls into one of these categories may be helpful:

>> **Physical (your body):** Is there something causing pain, discomfort, irritation? Are these factors making you want to avoid sexual situations? Are there thoughts or feelings that you have about your body (especially while it's going through some transitions) that cause you to steer clear of physical contact?

>> **Pharmaceutical (drug or medications):** Are you taking a medication that may have a side effect of decreasing your sexual interest? Many medications for high blood pressure or depression can have an influence on sexual thoughts and interest.

>> **Pathological (disease or illness):** Might you have a medical condition that causes fatigue, weakness, abdominal or pelvic pain or discomfort that would make sexual encounters uncomfortable or undesirable?

TIP

If you notice that your libido has dropped, and you want to get it back to where it was, work with your partner to make things better. Communicate and really talk about your situation. Do you have relationship problems? Does timing seem to play a part? Should you consider different techniques? You may need more foreplay, more stimulation, more lubricants, or different positions while your body and your relationship change.

A THEORY OF AROUSAL AND DESIRE IN WOMEN

In the 1960s, the famous sex research team of Masters and Johnson published work on the human sexual response cycle. They believed that both men's and women's sexual response could be divided into four phases: excitement, plateau, orgasm, and resolution. Their model was so influential that doctors used it to diagnose cases of sexual dysfunction all the way through the mid and late 1980s. But many sexual therapists and researchers realized that Masters and Johnson ignored one of the most important aspects of sexual behavior: that of desire. Without desire, people seemed to have little inclination to participate in sexual activity, and a lack of desire could easily extinguish whatever arousal existed. Also, Masters and Johnson's underlying implications seemed to suggest that intercourse and orgasm were the natural endpoints of a sexual interaction.

In 1999, a psychiatrist named Rosemary Basson introduced a newer model. She believed that most women see arousal and desire interchangeably. Many women are slow to feel sexually aroused, and only with that arousal do they begin to feel desire. Some women have no definite peak of arousal, and they need not reach orgasm to feel satisfied with a sexual encounter. Also, for many women, the desire for intimacy, not necessarily for sex, begins their sexual response cycle. For the women that Basson studied, it was the wish to connect intimately with a partner for a variety of positive reasons that caused them to enter the cycle of desire at any point, whether becoming receptive to sexual stimulation and intimacy, or actively seeking it out.

Sexual therapists and researchers view Basson's model as a circular one, with each phase stimulating and being stimulated by the preceding one. Unlike the Masters and Johnson model, Basson didn't use a linear model of Desire-->Arousal-->Orgasm. Instead, it consists of sexual and non-sexual elements that can affect each of the phases. This model (which you can see in the accompanying figure) suggests that these phases, and satisfaction with sexual encounters and relationships, are affected by satisfaction with relationships, self-image, and previous positive and negative sexual experiences. Note it is possible to enter this circular model at any point with the goal of sexual activity not necessarily being orgasm, but personal satisfaction.

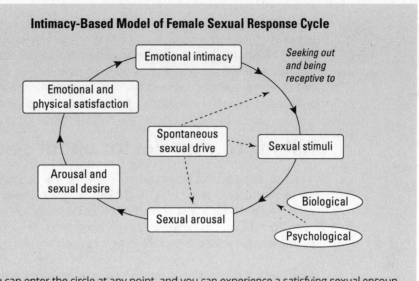

Intimacy-Based Model of Female Sexual Response Cycle

Emotional intimacy

Seeking out and being receptive to

Emotional and physical satisfaction

Spontaneous sexual drive

Sexual stimuli

Arousal and sexual desire

Biological

Psychological

Sexual arousal

You can enter the circle at any point, and you can experience a satisfying sexual encounter, even if you don't move through to some arbitrary endpoint.

How do I know if my libido is low?

The actual medical diagnosis for women who have low sex drive is called *hypoactive sexual desire disorder* (HSDD), and your doctor can give you a simple four-question survey to make the diagnosis:

>> In the past, was your level of sexual interest and desire good and satisfying to you?

>> Have you experienced a decline in your level of sexual interest/desire?

>> Do you feel bothered by your lack of sexual desire and interest?

>> Do you want your level of sexual desire and interest to increase?

If you answer "no" to any of these questions, your doctor likely won't diagnose you with HSDD. If you answer "yes" to all these questions, then the doctor should ask about one last subject. They want to ascertain whether your decrease in interest or desire relates to other factors, such as relationship issues, pain, medical or psychological conditions, recent childbirth or surgery, or a high level of stress and fatigue.

If you answer yes to all four screening questions, and no other reasons are identified, then your diagnosis likely is HSDD, and there are many things your doctor can suggest to help treat it.

REMEMBER

If identifiable physical or emotional factors seem to be contributing to your current lack of interest in sexual activity, then the treatment must address those factors. Physical pain or a poor relationship provide an obvious reason why you may want to avoid sex, and that reason may have nothing to do with your natural level of desire. You must address the pain, relationship issues, medical problems, or other factors before considering solutions to the problem of low libido.

Talking to your doctor about sex

Of course, to pursue an investigation into what's affecting your libido, you must talk to your doctor about it — don't wait for your doctor to bring it up! Many online surveys have asked women whether they talk to their doctors about this topic. Overwhelmingly, women say that they don't, for a variety of reasons. But the number one reason is that their doctors don't bring it up.

Many medical professionals ignore sexual issues when treating perimenopausal women:

>> They don't realize that you're experiencing a problem.

>> They feel embarrassed or uncomfortable when you mention a problem with sexual desire.

>> They may not have any good solutions or the latest information to offer.

   The majority of medical professionals know that sexual issues may occur during perimenopause, but they don't bring it up because they don't feel equipped to deal with it.

>> They have only a limited number of minutes in the room with you, so if *you* don't mention it, possibly neither will they.

WARNING

Switch doctors if this subject comes up, but your doctor doesn't seem to take it seriously, won't discuss it, or has no solutions to offer you (or at least a referral to a specialist who may be better able to help).

Like any other issue that interferes with your quality of life, this particular issue is important enough and specific enough to warrant hunting down a specialist. Most gynecologists, and certainly those that treat perimenopausal and menopausal women in their practices, should have a handle on how to evaluate and treat low libido; if you don't get a satisfactory work-up, keep looking.

Your gynecologist should gather the following information about your low libido:

>> **Take a thorough history of the problem.** They ask about all the things that could be affecting your desire: medical problems, changes in your

relationship, social situation, new medications that you may be taking, mental health issues, and stress. They ask about your history of desire, and if there was a time when lack of libido was *not* a problem.

>> **Ask about your level of distress.** Do you feel bothered by your current level of desire? (See the preceding section for discussion of the variations of a normal libido.)

Looking at the Factors That Can Mess with Your Libido

You can't fix libido issues by doing something as simple as taking a pill that can suddenly make you start to desire your partner (or anyone else). Even the studies that had women take Viagra to see its effects concluded that it didn't improve libido and desire in women in the way that it can improve performance in men. The female libido is multi-factorial, and looking at all the possible factors in play may give you, your doctor, and your partner a place to start.

Dropping estrogen levels

While you age, hormone levels fluctuate uncontrollably in perimenopause, and then they start to decline. The vagina has many estrogen *receptors* (molecules on the surface that bind to a specific substance — in this case, estrogen — and cause certain effects on that cell), and when estrogen levels begin to drop, the vaginal cells start to become thin and dry.

The medical community used to call this thinning and drying *atrophic vaginitis.* At some point, medical societies got tired of talking about women's vaginas as things that would just shrink and then disappear. So, they coined the term *genitourinary syndrome of menopause,* which starts to happen in perimenopause when your estrogen levels start to take a nosedive.

Genitourinary syndrome has many symptoms, and you don't have to have all of them to meet the criteria for a diagnosis:

>> Vaginal dryness

>> Vaginal burning

>> Genital itching

- >> Burning with urination (that's not caused by an infection)

- >> Urgency with urination

- >> Frequent urination

- >> Light bleeding after intercourse

- >> Discomfort with intercourse

- >> Decreased vaginal lubrication during sexual activity

- >> Shortening and tightness in the vaginal canal

If you're experiencing some these symptoms, you may respond by avoiding sex because of the discomfort that you know you'll likely experience during sexual activity, not necessarily because you lack desire.

REMEMBER

The simplest way to replace missing vaginal estrogen is to do just that — replace it. But discuss it with your doctor and have an evaluation first so that you can figure out whether using topical vaginal estrogen products is the right route for you. Not all women are candidates for using vaginal estrogen products because they may have certain medical conditions that preclude using it, and not all women want to use them because of a personal wish to avoid all hormone therapies.

Vaginal estrogen products

You can find many options when it comes to vaginal estrogen products. It's a personal choice which of these, if any, you want to use to make the vaginal tissue moister, thicker, and healthier. You and your doctor need to discuss and review your full medical history and symptoms to decide whether to use these treatments to relieve your vaginal dryness and pain.

REMEMBER

All vaginal estrogen products require a prescription in the U.S., and they come in many different formulations. They all treat just the local tissue, so they don't relieve any other symptoms of perimenopause, such as hot flashes or insomnia, because the doses are so low. Your insurance plan may cover some of these treatments, but not others.

Here's a list of the types of available vaginal estrogen products:

- >> **Estrogen cream:** You apply this product to the dry and thinning tissues by using an applicator or your finger. Usually, you use this cream twice a week at bedtime, although your doctor may recommend other dose regimens. Often, if the vaginal tissues are extremely dry, your doctor recommends that you use it every night for a week, and then go down to the two-to-three times a week usage.

>> **Estrogen tablets:** You place a tablet in your vagina at bedtime, also usually twice a week; these tablets melt at body temperature and are absorbed by your tissues. Again, you may need to start with a daily application at first, depending on how dry and thin your vaginal lining is.

>> **Estrogen suppositories:** Placed in the vagina at bedtime twice weekly; although sometimes, if the tissues are very dry, your doctor will recommend doing a jump-start routine of application every day for a week.

>> **Estrogen ring:** A silicone ring placed into the vagina and left in place for 90 days, emitting a small amount of estrogen all the time — in case you don't want to think about the daily or twice-weekly regimen.

>> **Prasterone:** A suppository made of a hormone called dehydroepiandrosterone (DHEA), which your adrenal glands normally produce. But when placed in the vagina, this suppository melts and, after being absorbed by the tissues, metabolizes into estrogen and testosterone (find out more in the section "Testosterone," later in this chapter). You use this suppository every night at bedtime, although some women find using it fewer times a week works well enough for them.

Estrogen product alternatives

Although estrogen is considered a first-line therapy for vaginal dryness and discomfort, if you can't or don't want to use vaginal estrogen (discussed in the preceding section), you have alternatives to consider if you want to bring back some moisture to those dry vaginal tissues:

VAGINAL MOISTURIZERS

These moisturizers can treat genitourinary syndrome, especially those moisturizers that contain hyaluronic acid (yes, the same stuff people use to lessen wrinkles). They reduce friction and temporarily improve vaginal dryness and pain during sexual activity. Usually, you apply them every two to three days. They adhere to the vaginal walls and hopefully provide some long-term relief.

VAGINAL LUBRICANTS

Provide temporary relief of vaginal symptoms at the time of sexual activity. They're divided into several categories:

>> *Water-based:* The most widely accessible type of lubricant, water-based lubricants cause fewer adverse effects than other types of lubricants, but you can't use them in water (the shower, bathtub, and so on) because the water will simply wash them away, and they evaporate quickly, so you may need to reapply them frequently.

>> *Silicone-based:* Waterproof, and thicker and more slippery than water-based lubricants. These lubricants last a long time and won't absorb into the skin, but you may find them a little harder to clean up than water-based lubricants.

>> *Oil-based:* Some women prefer to use natural oils, such as olive, coconut, and mineral oil, as lubricants. In general, these oils are moisturizing and thick, but they can potentially break down silicone-based condoms and might cause allergic reactions.

WARMING AND COOLING LUBRICANTS

You can find some specialty lubricants that have warming and/or cooling properties to them (a word of advice: try a little before you try a lot):

>> *Cooling lubes:* Typically contain peppermint, menthol, or other herbs that cause a chilling effect to the genital region.

>> *Warming gels:* May contain glycerin, capsaicin, or other herbal elements designed to cause a tingling or hot sensation.

The only way to know which moisturizers and lubricants work best for you is by doing a few test-runs to see which ones provide you with the best sense of comfort, relief, and enjoyment.

Vaginal or genital pain syndromes

Something other than dryness may be contributing to your discomfort during sex. Infections can cause vaginal or genital pain, and not just infections that you can contract from sexual partners. Bacterial vaginitis, yeast infections, and other infections can cause pain and discomfort during sex. If you have had symptoms of pain, discharge, burning, or itching please go get checked at a medical office so any infections can be properly treated.

Medical conditions can cause pain during sexual activity and, because of that pain, cause a decreased interest in sex. These conditions include:

>> **Endometriosis:** A condition in which the lining inside the uterus makes its way out of the uterus and into your pelvic cavity, implanting on your fallopian tubes, ovaries, intestines, or anywhere else in the pelvis. This condition can cause pain with sexual activity, and you and your doctor must diagnose and treat it so that you can regain comfort. Most women with endometriosis have a long history of painful periods, sometimes causing them to lose time from school or work.

- » **Ovarian cysts:** Every month at the time of ovulation (fewer than once a month in perimenopause because you're likely not ovulating every month anymore), a cyst or cysts can develop on or near the ovaries. Most ovarian cysts are just small fluid-filled growths, not dangerous and not of concern. But if they grow very large, twist or rupture, they can cause very painful conditions that worsen during sexual activity. Sometimes cysts can just be watched over time, but sometimes they require surgical removal.

- » **Skin conditions:** Aside from just general dryness on the skin of the vulva and genital area, skin conditions can appear and cause itching, burning, and pain. Your doctor can usually diagnose these skin conditions through history, exam, and sometimes a biopsy, and appropriate treatment can significantly diminish the pain that you may feel in the area. If your genital skin itches, burns, or just generally feels irritated or inflamed, a skin check is indicated.

- » **Herpes genitals:** A viral condition that causes periodic outbreaks on the skin of the genital area which can cause severe pain and open sore spots that may take days or weeks to heal and go away. This is a sexually transmittable virus that passes from person to person by skin-to-skin contact.

- » **Vaginismus:** A condition that causes the muscles of the vagina, perineum, and the surrounding area to tighten up and possibly spasm, making penetrative sexual activity painful, difficult, or impossible. You need to undergo some very specific treatments for this condition, and you usually need multiple types of these treatments. (More on this later in the chapter.)

- » **Vulvodynia:** A condition in which the nerves of the genital area become hypersensitive, making the slightest touch to the area painful. If you're diagnosed with this condition, you usually need to see a specialist in treating vulvar pain syndromes. (More on this later in the chapter.)

If any of these conditions may be causing your genital discomfort, address these sources of pain first if you want to possibly regain the desire for sex in the future.

WARNING

Both of the conditions vulvodynia and vaginismus may come with these symptoms:

- » Pain in the genital area (labia, clitoral area, urethra, at the vaginal opening, or inside the vagina) that happens with or without provocation (it may happen without sexual activity, just from clothing touching the area or from any pressure)

- » Pain and tight muscles at the opening to the vagina that prevents vaginal intercourse or the entry of a tampon into the vagina

These conditions require evaluation by a specialist in pelvic floor conditions — from a physician, nurse practitioner, or pelvic floor physical therapist who's familiar with pelvic and genital pain syndromes. You need more than vaginal estrogen or lubricants to relieve the extreme pain in these areas.

General medical conditions

Many health conditions can lead to a decrease in sex drive, so ask your doctor to evaluate you for these conditions if you're experiencing a decreased sex drive. Any of these conditions can lead to a decrease in interest in sex:

>> **Abnormal thyroid function:** Whether it's too low or too high, abnormal thyroid function seems to correlate with a lower libido in women. These conditions change the amount of sex hormones circulating in the body, which can then cause problems with sexual function. Studies have shown that correcting abnormal thyroid hormone levels is associated with an improvement in sexual function.

>> **Diabetes:** A condition in which levels of sugar in the bloodstream are too high. If diabetes is poorly managed (if the blood sugar levels are always higher than target ranges), consistent high blood sugar can cause damage to your blood vessels, preventing appropriate blood flow to the critical areas needed to help with libido: the brain and the genital region.

Also, when you have high blood sugar, it can interrupt your sleep, and many people suffer from fatigue during the day. Poor sleep and fatigue are definite libido killers.

>> **Heart disease:** Heart disease can cause a myriad of symptoms, including fatigue, stress, lowered energy, and other effects that lead to a lowered libido.

>> **High blood pressure:** Can cause low libido in the same way as diabetes: less blood flow to the critical areas (and potentially fatigue from interrupted sleep).

>> **Kidney disease:** Kidney disease can impact your libido in several ways, from effects of medications to the psychological strain of a chronic illness.

>> **Migraines:** The pain of migraines — severe and often throbbing, pulsating headaches — understandably lowers the libido.

If you already have any of these conditions, make sure that you treat them and have them under control with regular visits to your doctor. Not only can you improve your overall health, but you also may improve your sexual interest.

Psychological and social factors

For sexual interest and function to feel spontaneous and fulfilling, often, many other factors must be in place.

Libido is a complex intertwining of biological, psychological, social, and cultural influences. Figuring out the degree to which each of these factors influences your libido may help explain why your interest in sex may not be what you want it to be:

>> **Relationship issues:** Problems with communication, trust, or intimacy are among the most common causes of a decrease in sex drive.

>> **Stress:** Including stress from work, family, or life, in general (aging parents, kids leaving home, getting closer to retirement age). Stress can reduce your sex drive by taking your mind away from desire and focusing only on these stressful situations.

>> **Depression:** Low self-esteem, feelings of hopelessness, disappointment with the aging process and your aging body, and physical fatigue can lower your libido. Depression (along with lower estrogen levels) can cause an imbalance in the production of *neurotransmitters* (brain chemicals) that help regulate libido.

>> **Anxiety:** Can cause an increase in stress hormones (cortisol) and suppress the hormones that impact your sex drive.

>> **A history of sexual trauma:** To have healthy sexual desire and function, you usually need to establish trust and intimacy in relationships. A history of trauma often leaves victims feeling like they have no control, making future sexual relationships difficult or undesirable.

In your journey to locate and recover your feelings of sexual desire, make evaluating and treating any of these conditions a priority.

Medications

The list of medications that can impact libido is long. A history, including the timing of the medication and when the libido issues started in reference to the medication, can often uncover whether the lack of desire is truly associated with a particular medication. All these common medications can have an impact on your libido:

>> **Antidepressants:** Especially the class of medications called selective serotonin reuptake inhibitors (SSRIs) can have a well-known impact on sex drive because, to elevate levels of serotonin in your brain to help with depression and anxiety, they also cause a decrease in dopamine. Lower dopamine levels have been associated with a lower libido.

TIP

If you notice a marked difference in your libido after starting one of these medications, ask your doctor whether you can switch to another medication to treat your depression.

>> **High blood pressure medications:** Such as diuretics, beta blockers, and ACE inhibitors. These medications may cause a decrease in libido, which can lead people to go off their medications. Ask your doctor to substitute a medication that has less chance of causing sexual side effects, such as a medication in the category of angiotensin II receptor blockers (ARBs).

>> **Heart failure medication:** Beta blockers and diuretics, used to treat heart failure, can lower sexual interest and function.

>> **Opioid pain medications:** Studies show an association between long-term use of these pain medications and sexual dysfunction in women. Opioids likely interfere with the secretion of sex hormones, decreasing the interest in sexual activity and relationships.

>> **Anti-ulcer medications:** Chronic use of these drugs that fall into the category of histamine blockers (ranitidine, famotidine, and cimetidine) are linked with a decrease in testosterone and an increase in fatigue, both factoring into a lower libido.

>> **Seizure medications:** Such as phenytoin, carbamazepine, and phenobarbital, these medications have been shown to affect hormone levels. By decreasing hormone levels, they can influence a spontaneous desire for sex.

>> **Cholesterol medications:** Including rosuvastatin, atorvastatin, and simvastatin, these drugs may influence hormone levels, especially testosterone, which could have an impact on your libido.

If you think one of your medications is the culprit behind your decreased sexual desire, talk to your doctor. They may recommend stopping the medication or switching to a different one. Sometimes, you can use a second medication to deal with the sexual side effects of the first one.

Bringing Your Sexy Back: Ways to Restart or Ramp Up the Libido

If you don't have any of the issues discussed in the section "Looking at the Factors That Can Mess with Your Libido," earlier in this chapter — your relationship is good, you're attracted to your partner, and you don't have any medical conditions or take medications that can dampen your sex drive — but you still feel a lack of sexual interest, then you truly meet the definition of hypoactive sexual desire disorder (HSDD; check out the section "How do I know if my libido is low?" earlier in this chapter, for discussion of this medical issue). Unfortunately, medical science has a limited number of treatments available that have been shown to work for low libido in women.

Treatments for low libido include

>> **Information:** Really understanding sex, sexual behaviors, and sexual responses may help you to overcome anxieties about sexual function.

>> **Communication:** An open dialogue with your partner about your needs and concerns may also help overcome barriers to a healthy sex life. Talking to your partner about changes in your thoughts and your body may help you figure out strategies that can be mutually satisfying.

>> **Stress management:** Can improve how you respond to life stressors. Using techniques to reduce stress can help ease stress-induced symptoms, one of which may be low libido. Exercise, meditation, and journaling are forms of healthy stress management.

>> **Couples therapy:** May help you and your partner improve the overall quality of your relationship; you can figure out how to refine your relationship, work on resolving underlying problems, and find ways to increase intimacy and the expression of physical affection.

MEN HAVE VIAGRA — CAN'T I JUST TAKE SOMETHING?

Viagra, and medications like it, work by increasing the blood flow to the genital area, resulting in a longer, stronger erection and enhanced interest in sexual activity for men. Studies have been done to see if the same type of medication would have a similar stimulating effect for women's libido, but the results have been disappointing. That doesn't mean you don't have any medications that you can take to try to increase your level of sexual desire, but it does mean that nothing can do it *for sure*.

If you and your medical professional have ruled out all the other reasons for low libido, and you want to just try a supplement or a medication that may help, scientists have studied and tested a short list of some medications (see the section "Prescription medications" in this chapter). None of them have ever gotten as popular as Viagra, likely because women's libidos involve much more than just blood flow.

Supplements

You can purchase various supplements over the counter or online. There are no studies that prove they improve libido. They may contain

>> **Herbs and plant extracts:** Such as ashwagandha root, gingko biloba, rhodiola, maca root extract, and damiana

>> **Amino acids:** Such as L-arginine and L-citrulline

The marketing for these supplements may claim that they increase the amount of nitric oxide in the body, which supposedly helps with low libido. Viagra, the well-known erectile dysfunction treatment, works by increasing the amount of nitric oxide in the body, but studies have shown that women taking Viagra or medications like it don't have a notable improvement in their level of sexual desire.

Prescription medications

Only two medications are FDA-approved to treat symptoms of low libido in women:

>> **Flibanserin:** An oral medication that you take every day. It changes the activity of serotonin (a brain neurotransmitter), as well as other chemicals in the brain. It can take up to four weeks to work, and study results are mixed. It also can have some side effects such as low blood pressure and dizziness.

>> **Bremelanotide:** An on-demand injectable medication that you can use when the time is right. Within 45 minutes of injection, it increases sexual desire; it continues to work over the next 6 to 8 hours. You can use it up to eight times a month, but not more than once in 24 hours.

   Although we know that bremelanotide works on neurotransmitters in the brain, such as melanocortin, we don't know the actual mechanism by which this neurotransmitter level change leads to increased sexual desire. Nausea is a common side effect (not very sexy), and it may raise your blood pressure and heart rate.

Testosterone

Many people think that testosterone is the key to women's sexual desire. As you age, all hormone levels fluctuate and eventually decrease until, in menopause, they all disappear. So, it makes sense that if your hormones are changing and then decreasing, lower levels may cause a lower libido.

Although lower hormone levels in general may be responsible for decreasing sexual interest, the decrease in all hormones combined — estrogen, progesterone, and testosterone — mostly is what causes waning sexual desire. No studies show that lower testosterone levels alone cause a decrease in libido, nor that raising these levels absolutely raises libido. That being said, some studies show that women who take testosterone or who have higher levels of testosterone may also have higher libidos.

If you're wondering whether you might benefit from testosterone supplementation, find a medical practitioner who has had experience with all types of hormone replacement therapies. Possibly, the doctor will incorporate testosterone as part of a hormone replacement plan to help boost your libido. Studies (a relatively small number) have shown what levels of testosterone supplementation are safe in women.

WARNING

Testosterone isn't FDA-approved for women, and you face potential serious side effects if your doctor doesn't prescribe the proper doses or properly monitor your side effects and your testosterone levels. Many menopause and perimenopause healthcare specialists have experience with using testosterone in a hormone regimen and keep up to date with all the latest studies and information.

WARNING

Please don't buy testosterone online from questionable websites!

Using or taking testosterone in unmonitored and unchecked doses can result in

>> Acne

>> Aggressive behaviors

>> Heart or liver problems

>> Voice changes

>> Headaches

>> Excess body hair

>> Elevation in cholesterol levels

>> Vaginal bleeding

>> Cancers, including breast and uterine

Medical practitioners who have experience in prescribing testosterone can help you safely introduce this hormone into your perimenopausal hormone regimen, possibly enhancing your libido.

Specific Vaginal Pain Conditions

Earlier in the chapter I mentioned two conditions that can cause pain in the vaginal area, and they warrant further discussion. In the following sections we will look at these conditions, both of which carry symptoms that can be extremely uncomfortable and limiting in terms of activities, including sex.

Vulvodynia

This is the most common cause of painful intercourse and chronic pelvic pain in women who are still menstruating. This chronic unexplained pain in the area around the opening of the vagina can be so uncomfortable that some activities can feel unbearable.

Sitting for long periods of time, exercising, and having sex can be impossible. The pain may be described as burning, stinging, throbbing, stabbing, or soreness. Experts don't know what causes vulvodynia. Factors that might play a role include

>> Injury to the nerves of the vulva

>> Past chronic vaginal infections

>> Allergies

>> Hormonal changes

>> Skin reactions or inflammation

>> Muscle spasms or weakness in the pelvic floor muscles

>> Genetic factors

Without treatment, vulvodynia can affect mental health, relationships, and other aspects of your life. The condition is linked with anxiety and depression. It is also tied to less sexual desire, arousal, and enjoyment. A fear of having painful sex can cause spasms in the muscles around the vagina.

There are two types of vulvodynia, localized and generalized.

In cases of localized vulvodynia, the pain is isolated to one spot, like just at the opening to the vagina or just around the clitoral area. With generalized vulvodynia, the pain is not isolated to one spot. Instead, you may feel pain in different parts of the vulva and the vagina at different times. You may just feel generalized pain throughout the vulva.

Causes of vulvodynia

Vulvodynia can be provoked or unprovoked. In provoked vulvodynia, the pain is felt with touch or activity. With unprovoked vulvodynia you feel pain without any inciting factors.

Often, people with vulvodynia are also diagnosed with other common pain syndromes, including:

>> Fibromyalgia

>> Interstitial cystitis (painful bladder syndrome)

>> Irritable bowel syndrome

>> Temporomandibular disorder

Data suggests that people with vulvodynia are more likely to have higher levels of stress, histories of abuse, and certain behavioral health conditions including:

>> Anxiety

>> Depression

>> Post-traumatic stress disorder (PTSD)

Vulvodynia is diagnosed by ruling out other conditions that may be causing your pain. Your doctor will ask about your medical, sexual, and surgical history. They will also ask about your symptoms, including the location of the pain, what the pain feels like, when, and how badly the vulvar area hurts.

Tests and procedures used to diagnose vulvodynia may include:

>> **Physical exam:** Your provider will inspect the vulvar area and perform a pelvic exam, including a possible exam with a speculum to assess your vagina and cervix. She will also evaluate the pelvic floor including the muscles to identify painful areas.

>> **Cotton swab test (point pressure testing):** Your provider may brush a cotton swab gently over various parts of the vulva, asking when and where this contact feels painful. This is especially helpful in locating pain in the area between the vagina and the urethra.

>> **Swabs to test for infection:** These tests can rule out pain that is caused from infections, like sexually transmitted infections and other bacterial and yeast infections.

Biopsy. Sometimes specific areas of the vulvar skin need to be biopsied to make a diagnosis or to rule out other conditions.

Treating vulvodynia

Vulvodynia treatment usually takes an extended period of time. Finding the right treatment or combinations of treatments to bring pain relief sometimes involves trial and error.

Treatments may include:

>> **Topical medications:** Creams and ointments that numb the vulvar area (anesthetics) can be used for pain relief. Topical neuromodulator medications can also be used to stabilize or relieve irritated nerves. Hormonal creams containing estrogen and progesterone can also be part of a treatment plan.

>> **Oral medications:** Antidepressants and anti-seizure medications can be used to reduce nerve pain.

>> **A nerve block:** An injection can be used to prevent pain signals from traveling from the nerves of the vulvar area to the brain.

>> **Physical therapy:** This can be used to loosen muscle tension in the pelvic floor. The muscles, ligaments, and connective tissue in the pelvis may spasm and contract involuntarily, and physical therapy can help relieve these spasms. Treatment may also involve stretching, lengthening, and strengthening weak pelvic floor muscles.

>> **Surgery:** A surgery called a vestibulectomy can be helpful for people with localized vulvodynia whose pain hasn't improved with more conservative treatments. During this procedure the tissue that feels painful is removed.

>> **Counseling:** Individual counseling, couple's counseling, or sex therapy may help improve the areas of your life impacted by the pain of vulvodynia, especially for improvement in sexual relationships.

It is unknown whether vulvodynia will ever completely resolve. If you have persistent pain in your vulvar area, schedule an appointment with your doctor. Treatment may require a team-based approach with multiple modalities. The sooner you can connect with multiple resources, the sooner you can experience relief.

Vaginismus

This is the body's automatic reaction to the fear of some or all types of vaginal penetration. Whenever vaginal penetration is attempted, the vaginal muscles reflexively tighten on their own. This condition does not necessarily affect your ability to become sexually aroused or to enjoy other types of sexual contact, but intercourse is often impossible.

Sometimes vaginismus develops later in life, sometimes after years without having any problems. Spasms or discomfort may occur at any time an attempt is made at vaginal penetration. Healthcare experts aren't sure why some people experience vaginismus. Factors that may contribute to it include:

>> Anxiety disorders

>> Childbirth injuries such as vaginal tears

>> Prior surgery or damage to the tissues

>> Fear of sex or negative feelings about sex due to cultural issues or prior trauma or sexual abuse

Vaginismus is diagnosed with a thorough history and a pelvic/vaginal exam. Your provider may need to apply an anesthetic (numbing) cream in order to perform an adequate exam.

Treatment focuses on reducing the reflex of your muscles that cause them to tense up involuntarily. Treatments also address the anxieties or fears that can contribute to vaginismus.

Topical therapies, pelvic floor physical therapy, and vaginal dilator therapy may all be needed to treat vaginismus. Dilator therapy uses tube-shaped devices to stretch the vaginal tissues to become more comfortable with and less sensitive to vaginal penetration.

Therapies, like cognitive behavioral therapy and sex therapy, can also help in the treatment of vaginismus.

Many people with vaginismus no longer experience pain after treatment. Successful treatment takes time and often utilizes a combination of therapies. If vaginal penetration seems impossible or is always painful, seek medical care for a proper exam and diagnosis.

3

Prioritizing Mental Health and Wellbeing

Understand how perimenopause can play with your mind.

Pay attention to your mental health and wellbeing.

Get enough rest and practice other acts of self-care.

Chapter **8**

Brain Changes: What to Expect and What to Do When the Fog Rolls In

Have you ever realized in the middle of talking with someone that you're having trouble following the conversation? Or that you can't find the right words for something that you were trying to explain? Or that you even forgot the name of the person you're talking to? These occurrences happen to everyone occasionally, but in midlife, you may find that this kind of forgetfulness starts to happen with worrisome regularity.

Women in midlife commonly complain of poor concentration, trouble remembering words or concepts, and a general feeling of brain fog. You may be worried about the implications of these changes: "Do they mean I'm heading toward dementia? Can I stop these memory changes before I lose all of my brain function?" You can find these memory lapses annoying, but they don't necessarily mean that you have Alzheimer's disease or any other form of dementia — or that you're going to develop one.

In this chapter, you can explore how hormonal changes that occur during perimenopause — from fluctuation to absence — affect your brain. This chapter provides you with information about how the changes in perimenopause affect brain function: everything from changes in blood flow to the brain, to the hormonal effects on your brain chemistry. You can also find out about ways to slow down this process or try to halt it altogether.

What's Taken Over Your Brain?

The brain works kind of like a big computer. It's roughly the size of two clenched fists, with folds and crevices on its surface. The brain has various sections, each with its own function and specialty. The brain requires a steady flow of oxygen, sugar (*glucose*), and other nutrients to work properly. The brain performs its functions by sending and receiving chemical and electrical signals via nerves that run throughout the body. The brain interprets these signals, allowing for the coordination of thought, emotion, behavior, movement, and sensation.

A complicated series of connections controls everything that happens in your body, and memory lapses or fuzzy thinking can signal that the connections aren't running so smoothly or working properly. When we learn something — even something as simple as someone's name — we form connections between the nerve cells (called *neurons*) in the brain. These connections form new circuits, creating a map in the brain. Anything that disrupts these connections, or these maps, can interrupt your brain while it tries to form memories.

During perimenopause, you may experience neurological changes that can concern, confuse, and frustrate you.

TECHNICAL STUFF

Many scientists believe that brain fog has something to do with the hormonal changes that take place during perimenopause. During the menopausal transition, women often start to experience poor concentration or brain fog, with hormonal changes as the likely culprit. *Brain fog* is loosely defined as a state of mind characterized by confusion, forgetfulness, a lack of focus, and poor mental clarity. You may find brain fog particularly distressing if you always felt that you had quite a sharp memory and impressive brain function in your younger years.

Levels of estrogen and progesterone vary widely during this time, and these ricochets can cause all kinds of lapses in brain function. Your brain doesn't operate at its best during perimenopause for a couple of reasons:

>> **Blood flow:** When estrogen levels are high, the brain gets enough of it to keep blood vessels open and maintain good blood flow to the brain, allowing sharp thinking and a sense of well-being. Estrogen exerts a positive effect on the lining of blood vessels, keeping them healthy and able to allow blood, carrying oxygen, to reach its destination.

While perimenopause-related hormonal ups and downs continue, they can lead to more frequent memory slips and worsening mental function. When estrogen levels decline with age and then hit zero in menopause, blood vessel health and blood flow continue to diminish.

>> **Poor sleep:** Lower hormone levels can cause night sweats and hot flashes, resulting in interrupted sleep. Poor sleep can contribute to cognitive decline because sleep that's not restorative or deep enough can have a detrimental effect on daytime brain function, concentration, and activity. Waking up tired is a setup for a day where you not only don't feel sharp, but probably would just rather go back to sleep.

The brain, when impacted by hormonal changes or absence, plays a big role in many of the recognized symptoms of perimenopause. The following sections talk about some symptoms that you may not have considered brain-related.

Nearly impossible multitasking

In your younger days, you may have been an accomplished juggler. Maybe you had to handle a multitude of simultaneous responsibilities while you balanced job duties, relationships, raising children, and household chores. When multitasking, the brain needs to switch back and forth between the parts of the brain that code for short-term memory and the part that's activated when you need to pay attention to something new. Younger brains can switch quickly between different neurological networks; but for older brains, the switch takes more time (if it happens at all). While we get older, interruptions and distractions can cause difficulty with concentration and the quality of memory. Changes in hormones in midlife can cause this inability to multitask, forcing you to focus on only one thing at a time.

TIP

Bear in mind that the idea of multitasking might be a myth — some studies show that when our brain is constantly switching gears to bounce back and forth between tasks, we become less efficient at all of them and more likely to make mistakes. So maybe focusing on one thing at a time is better!

Regulating body temperature

A part of the brain called the hypothalamus regulates our internal body temperature. It constantly checks our body temperature and compares it to normal body temperature (approximately 98.6 degrees Fahrenheit; 37 degrees Celsius). If your temperature is too low, the hypothalamus stimulates the body to make more heat and, if the temperature is too high, it signals the body to eliminate that heat.

In perimenopause, when you have sometimes drastic fluctuations in hormone levels, the brain gets a signal that your body's hotter than it actually is. In an attempt to release the excess heat, it causes your body to sweat (because sweat evaporates from the skin and cools the body down). This signal misfire can happen multiple times a day (and night), when the brain gets incorrect signals due to wide fluctuations in estrogen levels.

Snoozing soundly — or not

The perimenopausal shift in hormone levels can have some dramatic effects on your body's biology. *Melatonin* is a hormone that is released naturally by your brain into your bloodstream nightly to produce regular cycles of sleep. Estrogen plays a role in stimulating the production and the release of melatonin. When estrogen levels start to decline, your brain releases less melatonin, leading to poor sleep — trouble both falling asleep and staying asleep.

Research has shown that over 50 percent of women report some type of ongoing insomnia in the years leading up to their final menstrual period. Poor sleep can affect every aspect of your life. (See Chapter 11.)

Dealing with forgetfulness

Sixty to 70 percent of women in midlife report some changes in their memory, such as forgetting things or having difficulty mastering new tasks. The fluctuations in hormone levels that occur in perimenopause could have something to do with these brain issues.

Forgetting can happen if the brain doesn't reinforce a memory frequently enough or long enough to store it. Estrogen supports blood flow to the brain, and the brain needs constant blood flow to make and store memories.

Navigating mood shifts

Brain chemicals, also called *neurotransmitters,* are responsible for stable moods and emotional well-being. Serotonin, dopamine, norepinephrine, and Gamma-aminobutyric acid (GABA) are neurotransmitters that are made and released by the nerve cells of the brain (called *neurons*). Neurotransmitters regulate many body functions, including emotional and mental well-being. Estrogen has an impact on the production of some neurotransmitters, especially serotonin; and serotonin's presence (or absence) has an impact on moods. When you have unstable estrogen levels, you also have unstable serotonin levels, resulting in the mood swings of perimenopause.

GETTING OFF THE HORMONE ROLLER COASTER

Although many women complain about menopause, at least menopause is a time where the ovaries are producing no hormones whatsoever, so you don't have to deal with swings or fluctuations in hormone levels. Research has shown (as has talking to many women, anecdotally) that the period of time preceding menopause, the five to nine years leading up to that last menstrual period, are worse in many ways than being in menopause because fluctuating hormones wreak more havoc than absent hormones.

Improving Cognitive Function in Perimenopause and Beyond

I can offer one reassuring thing about perimenopausal brain changes: Most research shows that these changes are temporary. The changes in your brain function that you associate with perimenopause likely improve after all these hormonal fluctuations stop and you're safely in menopause.

Although not everyone experiences memory lapses, if you do, you may find the experience scary. When you notice that you're increasingly forgetful and suddenly struggling to complete tasks, it's hard not to think about your aunt who has dementia or your neighbor whom officers found wandering outside at night. Just because you experience the occasional lost car keys (or sometimes even forget where your car is parked) doesn't mean you're headed for dementia. If you find it difficult to retain information, despite writing endless to-do lists, you can follow the recommendations in this section to get a handle on your perimenopausal brain.

If you go through this list of recommendations to assist your brain function, but your hormonal swings (and the moods that they may cause and the sleep disruptions that simply don't stop) are still sabotaging your ability to think clearly (and to remember your keys and your appointments), you have ways to stabilize those hormonal fluctuations.

When you're going through perimenopause, absolutely discuss hormone therapy with your doctor and consider it as a solution for symptoms that interfere with your quality of life.

Although doctors don't prescribe hormones specifically to address the issue of brain fog (no one yet has conducted studies that show taking hormones can reduce your chances of dementia, improve your memory, or even help you remember where you parked). However, studies do show that women who use hormone replacement for bothersome hot flashes and night sweats may also see improvement in concentration and memory. (See Chapter 6.)

Whether you and your doctor decide to try one of the many types of hormonal contraception available to most perimenopausal women or you work with a hormone specialist to see how menopausal hormone therapy (MHT) can help, eliminating the hills and valleys of estrogen and progesterone production may help you put your brain back on the road to solving those puzzles and helping that fog to lift.

Even if you feel confident that perimenopause, and the hormonal changes that go along with it, are causing your discouraging changes in brain function, go through this checklist before deciding that you have a hormonal problem that has a hormone solution. Brain fog and memory issues can be caused by many things, and the conditions and habits in this list may factor in — and you (and your doctor) don't want to miss them:

>> **Check for medical conditions that can cause a deterioration in brain function.** Diabetes, thyroid dysfunction, high blood pressure, heart disease, and some autoimmune diseases can decrease the amount of blood flow to the brain, causing symptoms of brain fog and poor concentration. Have a full physical exam, possibly get some blood work, and discuss your concerns about your brain function with your doctor.

>> **If you smoke, quit.** Among the many reasons to stop smoking (if you reach perimenopause still attached to this bad habit), include the fact that smoke, and the carbon monoxide that smoking produces, restricts oxygen flow to the brain. Neurons in the brain that are deprived of oxygen will slowly die, and no one can revive them.

>> **Get enough deep, restorative sleep.** Although many women have trouble sleeping during the perimenopausal period, waking up in the middle of the night is likely to affect your brain's ability to function. Improving your sleep during this time boosts mood, energy levels, and concentration. (See Chapter 11 for more information on dealing with the sleep changes that come with perimenopause.)

>> **Eat a healthy diet.** The foods that you eat have important links to healthy brain function. Researchers have found evidence that whole grains, green leafy vegetables, legumes, monounsaturated fats and oils, and Omega-3 fatty acids (such as those you find in fatty fish) all support healthy brain function. Researchers also connect limiting trans fats, processed foods, high sugar foods, and sugary drinks to better cognitive function. (Flip to Chapter 13 for a discussion on diet.)

>> **Limit alcohol consumption.** Alcohol's effect on the brain greatly depends on how much you drink. Although a minimal amount of alcohol may have some benefit, heavier drinking has more negative effects, especially on the brain. Drinking may

- Trigger hot flashes

- Interfere with the brain's communication pathways

- Contribute to feelings of anxiety and depression

Alcohol is a central nervous system depressant; it slows down the system, causing you to speak, think, and act more slowly. Moderate levels of alcohol over a long period of time can make it more difficult to learn and to hold onto knowledge.

>> **Exercise your body.** Get yourself moving! Aerobic exercise (exercise that makes you sweat and gets your heart pumping) boosts blood flow to your brain and boosts the size of the part of the brain involved in verbal memory and learning (the *hippocampus*). Physical activity can boost memory, improve thinking, and lower dementia risks.

A 2022 study found that older adults who remain active have higher levels of brain proteins that enhance connections between neurons, which in turn improve their memory and boost cognition.

>> **Exercise your mind.** Nothing exercises and challenges the mind like puzzles. Crossword puzzles, number puzzles, word puzzles, jigsaw puzzles — they all provide opportunities to stimulate the mind and improve brain function. Puzzles that require you to look for patterns, to pay attention to details, and to rely on memory can help the brain to change, reorganize, and create new pathways for learning. Traveling, trying new foods and recipes, or learning a new language or a new skill all help improve and stimulate your midlife brain function.

READ THE LABEL: MEDICATIONS THAT CAN ADD TO THE FOG

Be very careful with medications. Many medicines affect brain function, especially medications that you may take to treat insomnia, anxiety, or depression, as well as sedatives and opiate pain medications. Avoid the PM versions of over-the-counter pain medications, and talk with your doctor about any medications that contain any of the following drugs, grouped by the condition that they treat.

Allergies:

- Diphenhydramine (Benadryl)
- Promethazine (also for nausea)

Anxiety:

- Alprazolam (Xanax)
- Amitriptyline (also for insomnia and nerve pain)
- Diazepam (Valium)
- Lorazepam (Ativan)
- Nortriptyline (Pamelor; also for depression, insomnia, and nerve pain)
- Paroxetine (Paxil; also for depression)

Bladder issues (overactive bladder, urgency, leakage):

- Oxybutynin (Oxytrol)
- Tolterodine (Detrol)

Depression:

- Nortriptyline (Pamelor; also for anxiety, insomnia, and nerve pain)
- Paroxetine (Paxil; also for anxiety)

Dizziness:

- Meclizine (for dizziness and vertigo)
- Scopolamine (for dizziness, motion sickness, and vertigo)

Insomnia:

- Amitriptyline (also for anxiety and nerve pain)

- Eszopiclone (Lunesta)

- Nortriptyline (Pamelor; also for anxiety, depression, and nerve pain)

- Temazepam (Restoril)

- Zaleplon (Sonata)

- Zolpidem (Ambien)

Nerve pain:

- Amitriptyline (also for anxiety and insomnia)

- Nortriptyline (Pamelor; also for anxiety, depression, and insomnia)

Pain:

- Codeine

- Cyclobenzaprine (also for muscle relaxation)

- Hydrocodone

- Hydromorphone

- Morphine

- Oxycodone

- Tramadol

Psychiatric conditions:

- Aripiprazole (Abilify; for bipolar disorder and schizophrenia)

- Risperidone (Risperdal; for autism, bipolar disorder, and schizophrenia)

This list is by no means all-inclusive, and if you find that you're taking one of the medications listed in this sidebar while dealing with compromised brain function, you may want to consult with a healthcare professional to discuss alternatives to these medications for treating your medical conditions.

GIVING YOUR MEMORY A LITTLE SUPPORT

I have a 52-year-old patient who has seen me for the past six years. I can tell that her memory has gotten worse over time. She began to forget treatment plans that we discussed, referrals I made to other physicians — and one year, she even forgot to get her mammogram. We discussed these changes and came to the conclusion that she could benefit from some hormone replacement, specifically for her night sweats (which were waking her four or five times a night, so she was sleeping poorly). But we also came up with a reminder system for her to use: She brought in a notebook to her appointments, and I would print out anything that we discussed at her visit (including the date of the discussion), which she then taped into her book. She just needed that physical reminder to look at every day, and she never forgot our discussions or her prescriptions again.

Were her memory problems resolved by the hormones, better sleep, or my notebook solution? I think that some combination of all three provided my patient with the memory boost she needed.

Chapter **9**

Mental Health Changes: You're Not Imagining It

During reproductive years, you will usually become accustomed to your own hormonal rhythm. There may be a time of the month that you feel happy; a time of the month when you feel more anxious, stressed, or down. When this rhythm is disrupted during perimenopause, one of the results may be mood changes.

Mood swings, short-term memory loss, and difficulty thinking straight are all common complaints from midlife women. But if you find yourself feeling down or anxious, or emotional a majority of your days, it may be time to evaluate whether hormone swings are responsible for mood swings, or may this be something else?

A 50-year-old woman came to see me. She said she went to her primary care doctor and told him, "I don't know what's wrong. I'm crying all the time, I'm exhausted, and I can't sleep." Her doctor said, "I think you need to go see your gynecologist." Smart doctor!

Although weepiness for seemingly no reason may not seem like a gynecological affair, hormone shifts are directly tied to emotional fluctuation. While we enter perimenopause, such ups and downs can catch us by surprise — but these shifts can be completely normal.

Some women suffer from premenstrual syndrome (PMS) their entire reproductive lives, whereas others seem completely unaffected by the bodily changes taking place while they experience the different phases of their menstrual cycles. But hormones play some role in mental and emotional well-being for almost everyone. In your midlife years, whatever emotional stability you have may vanish. The smallest change in plans or an off-hand comment (often by someone you barely know) can send you into an emotional tailspin. Maybe you feel an uneasiness or irritability about everyday things that you haven't felt since adolescence. You're not alone.

In this chapter, you can start to figure out whether these changes in your emotional state are normal and expected, whether they have some connection to your changing hormones, and how to differentiate them from severe and/or serious mental health problems that may require a different and specific pathway for treatment and relief.

Not Just in Your Head: Your Emotions Really Are "All Over the Place"

One of the most common but least understood emotional changes during perimenopause are those infamous *mood swings*. You may feel calm, with a sense of well-being — even happiness — one minute; and then, seemingly without a trigger, you feel sad, depressed, and gloomy. You may snap at your spouse or your kids when they ask a simple question, such as, "Are you okay?" These mood swings may happen only occasionally, without impacting your life or your relationships with your family and friends. Or they may start to affect your relationships with family and friends.

But if these mood swings happen on the regular, and you continue to have drastic shifts from sad, to happy, and back down again, talk to your physician or mental health expert. Certain conditions that require medication and therapy may start to appear in midlife and aren't just normal perimenopausal changes.

Anxiety

Anxiety is intense, excessive, and persistent worry. It may be a normal reaction in stressful situations, but it can cause negative physical symptoms. If public speaking or pulling onto a very busy super-highway causes you to feel sweaty, with a fast heartbeat and rapid breathing, you may have *situational anxiety*. During perimenopause, you can experience anxiety for a variety of reasons.

Perimenopause is a time of rapid swings in hormone levels. If you happen to be a woman who's sensitive to these hormonal changes, it can feel just like situational anxiety. These hormonal changes can also cause a fast heartbeat, sweating, and rapid breathing. Women who have high stress levels in everyday life, and who have severe hot flashes and sleep disturbances during perimenopause, tend to have more feelings of anxiety.

They may be most aware of these sensations in the mornings because cortisol, also called the "stress hormone," is higher in the mornings for people that are under a lot of stress. Waking up with feelings of stress and worry may indicate an anxiety disorder. Estrogen and progesterone levels can also be low at certain times of the month, like right before you are about to get a period. Lower levels of estrogen can also cause a feeling of anxiety in the mornings.

TIP

If you're experiencing anxiety, you have several options — from hormone therapy to yoga — that may alleviate symptoms. The section "Addressing the Ups and Downs of Your Emotions," later in this chapter, offers some suggestions.

If you're also experiencing other symptoms of perimenopause, such as hot flashes and sleep disturbances, your physician may recommend a trial of some type of hormone therapy to stabilize your hormones and eliminate some of the swings.

If a fair trial of hormone therapy (usually several months) doesn't relieve your anxiety symptoms, you can try many other ways to address those symptoms. Prescription medications for depression and for anxiety may treat debilitating anxiety symptoms by changing the balance of certain brain chemicals, called *neurotransmitters,* which can exert a stabilizing and calming effect on your heart rate, breathing, and racing thoughts.

Again, if your doctor recommends these medications, have a detailed discussion of the risks and benefits with them, and give the medication some time to work. If the medication doesn't help, discuss a different dose or a different medication with your doctor. Psychotherapy and cognitive behavioral therapy (CBT) have both proven effective for helping with anxiety in the perimenopausal period. Mind-body and exercise techniques may also help relieve the symptoms of perimenopausal stress and anxiety.

Taking care of your overall health prior to entering perimenopause can also help you prepare for the possible onset of perimenopausal anxiety. If you realize that you don't have the best coping skills, please make use of the many books and online resources (see Appendix B).

During perimenopause, you may face increased stress in the form of work deadlines, family drama, aging parents, children moving away or moving back in, changes in relationships, death, divorce . . . the list is endless. And fluctuating hormones at the very same time can make coping seem impossible.

Your coping abilities may also be subject to wide swings. Sometimes, you cope. And sometimes, the anxiety may seem to be getting the better of you. (Chapter 5 goes into the many coping methods that will serve you in perimenopause and beyond.)

Depression

When estrogen levels fluctuate during the perimenopausal transition, it causes levels of brain chemicals, called *neurotransmitters*, to fluctuate, as well. Some of these chemical transmitters are serotonin, norepinephrine, and dopamine. They play a direct role in your mood, and when they're present and in balance, you usually have a feeling of calm.

When hormones, especially estrogen and progesterone, are higher or lower than previously or are rapidly changing, this imbalance can inhibit the ability of these neurotransmitters to be produced and to act effectively, which can result in mood swings, anxiety, and depression.

Depression is a major medical illness that can affect how you feel and how you think, and it can lead to a variety of physical and emotional problems. You may wonder, "If I'm sad, does that mean I have depression?" But depression is a specific, serious set of symptoms that can't be attributed to any other medical condition.

TIP

The symptom list is long, and most people have some of these symptoms some of the time. If your symptoms seem situational (i.e., being sad at the loss of a friend, or a problem at work), and are temporary, it does not mean you have depression. If the symptoms last long (i.e., longer than a month or two), seem not to be related to a specific event, and are compromising your day-to-day function and quality of life, that may require an evaluation. These symptoms may include

>> Fatigue

>> Lack of energy

>> Inattentiveness

>> Lack of interest in activities that you used to enjoy

>> Feelings of worthlessness, hopelessness, or helplessness

>> Tearfulness for no apparent reason

>> Sleeping more than usual, but not feeling rested and not wanting to get out of bed

>> Change in appetite — usually eating less, but sometimes eating more or erratically

>> Slowed movements or speech

>> Difficulty concentrating or making decisions

>> Thoughts of self-harm, death, or suicide

To be diagnosed with depression, your doctor will try to rule out medical problems that may cause these symptoms (such as thyroid abnormalities, neurological problems, or vitamin deficiencies). The symptoms must continue for at least two weeks and represent a change from your prior level of functioning to qualify as clinical depression.

Often, women who have no prior history of depression may begin to experience depression in perimenopause. Events that may occur around the time of perimenopause — such as divorce, loss of a job, death of a family member, or medical diagnoses — may trigger depression.

If you have felt these feelings of sadness and depression for a long time — months or years even, but have only recently sought help — your doctor will take a detailed history and make some suggestions as to how to treat what may be an ongoing depressive episode.

Certain factors increase your risk for depression in midlife, including

>> **Family history of depression:** When there are family members who have been diagnosed with depression, there may be a familial or a genetic link as to why you may feel these symptoms as well.

>> **Prior history of domestic violence or sexual abuse:** Feeling helpless or out of control in a relationship leads to feelings of depression.

>> **Severe perimenopausal symptoms, such as hot flashes or poor sleep:** These can leave you feeling fatigued all day and unable to cope with life's stressors.

>> **Social isolation:** Having no one that can listen to your symptoms or feelings of dissatisfaction can make you keep these feelings to yourself, causing a build-up of strong emotions. This can lead to a feeling of hopelessness.

>> **Low self-esteem:** If you feel you have no tools available for you to work out feelings of sadness, it may cause you to feel you deserve these feelings and there is nothing that can make you feel any better.

- >> **Sedentary lifestyle:** Exercise is a well-known antidote to feelings of sadness or emotional pain. While exercise cannot change your social situation, it changes the levels of stress hormones in your brain and can improve your sense of control and coping capabilities.

- >> **Smoking:** Some smokers say they do it because it relieves their stress and anxiety. But studies show that when people stop smoking they generally have lower levels of depression and anxiety. Evidence suggests that the beneficial effect of stopping smoking on symptoms of anxiety and depression can equal that of taking anti-depressants.

- >> **History of post-partum depression:** Women who have had depression that was diagnosed in the postpartum period (up to 6 months after giving birth). There is evidence to suggest that women with postpartum depression have an increased vulnerability to future depressive episodes.

REMEMBER

Also, have you thought — really thought — about how you feel about moving toward menopause and aging, in general? May women have negative thoughts about aging; combined with some of the risk factors in the preceding list and the fluctuating hormones of perimenopause, you may inevitably feel somewhat sad about this part of life.

But depression doesn't have to be a part of your life during perimenopause. Discuss treatments for depression and some preventative measures with your doctor. People who seek help for their depression are likely to find relief.

Because depression and perimenopause have a complex relationship, only a visit with your doctor — where the two of you thoroughly evaluate your history, symptoms, and any physical and mental changes — can determine which pathway to follow to treat new-onset perimenopausal depression.

Some medications that treat hot flashes also may treat depression (certain serotonin-increasing medications); these medications have their own side effects and risks, so your doctor and you need to decide what course of treatment makes the most sense for you. But many women do find relief with these medications.

Of course, you can also try a variety of home remedies for dealing with depression, such as regular exercise, proper restorative sleep, mindfulness techniques, breathing exercises, and certain supplements. See "Addressing the Ups and Downs of Your Emotions," later in this chapter.

Irritability

Seventy percent of women describe feeling irritable at some point during their perimenopausal transition. It manifests itself as a lack of patience and a low tolerance level for things that never used to set them off. Some women feel that the other symptoms of perimenopause that they're experiencing, such as poor sleep and inability to concentrate, contribute to this feeling of irritation. And some report feeling irritated or sad for no clear reason.

If you feel that, in this life stage, you're less patient, more irritable, and shorter tempered, you can try to develop some skills to give you relief — before these feelings escalate and become perimenopausal rage. (I go into that form of anger in the following section.) If you get irritable only temporarily, and in relation to a particular situation, consider these methods of coping:

>> Remove yourself from an upsetting situation.

>> Seek a counselor or therapist.

>> Find a trusted friend with whom you can discuss your feelings.

>> Do something that you enjoy, such as exercise, listen to music, watch a television show.

But if the frustrations and irritability continue, even when you've attempted one or several coping methods, your moods may connect directly to hormonal swings, an imbalance in neurotransmitters, or other diagnosable medical conditions that your doctor can help you uncover by doing a thorough evaluation.

Anger

Some women experience a surprising emotion that they never felt prior to midlife. They begin to experience deep anger, also called *perimenopausal rage.* This type of anger may feel different from ordinary anger or frustration. It can escalate from a feeling of relative stability to a feeling of intense resentment and irritability in a matter of moments. You may recognize that suddenly you don't have as much patience as you used to have, and family or friends may notice the same.

As with many other perimenopausal symptoms, this anger and rage occur for a chemical reason — the balance between estrogen and serotonin. When your ovaries produce estrogen in adequate amounts, your brain also releases serotonin in adequate amounts, helping to create a sense of calm and stability.

When you have wide swings in the production of estrogen, as well as estrogen levels that are generally declining over time, serotonin production also becomes unreliable, and you may lose that sense of calm. Women in perimenopause often feel like they're functioning on their last nerve, and one unexpected or triggering event may cause a sudden and unbalanced sense of irritability that may quickly escalate to rage.

What can you do to regain control of these moods? Women are generally the great suppressors. They suppress anger and other feelings so as not to inconvenience anyone else. *Self-silencing*, or not finding ways to acknowledge and express your anger, can be an unhealthy habit that can put you at higher risk for depression.

WARNING

Some lifestyle habits — such as smoking, not drinking enough water throughout the day, and consuming a lot of caffeine — can trigger anxiety and irritability, leading to bouts of anger and rage.

Identifying the triggers that lead to your episodes can go a long way toward prevention. Knowing that perimenopause is a time of escalated emotions can help you deal with frustrations by taking a step back, evaluating the situation, and realizing that you can take certain actions at a later, less emotional, time so that you can hopefully prevent similar episodes in the future.

Finding outlets, such as vigorous exercise, gardening, painting, and writing (even journaling about your experiences) all provide you with good ways to save space for yourself. Self-care is so important during this time of great upheaval, and taking the time out for yourself may move you toward an overall calm and fewer irritating or angry episodes.

TECHNIQUES TO PRACTICE THAT HELP MANAGE FEELINGS OF ANGER IN PERIMENOPAUSE (AND BEYOND)

Anger management can be particularly beneficial during perimenopause, when hormonal fluctuations can lead to mood swings, irritability, and increased susceptibility to anger. Here are some tips for managing feelings of anger:

Recognize the signs of anger: Pay attention to physical cues like tensed muscles, increased heart rate, and rapid breathing, and recognize emotional signs like irritability, frustration, and a strong desire to retaliate.

Take a pause: When you feel anger rising, take a step back. Remove yourself from the situation, if possible. Count to ten or take deep breaths to give yourself time to cool down.

Practice deep breathing: Inhale slowly through your nose, hold for a few seconds, and then exhale slowly through your mouth. This helps to calm your nervous system and bring your emotions under control.

Avoid negative self-talk: Replace harsh self-criticism with positive affirmations. Remind yourself that it's okay to feel angry, but it's important to respond in a healthy way.

Find a healthy outlet for release: Engage in physical activities like jogging, yoga, or even a brisk walk to release pent-up energy. Or practice a creative hobby, like painting, writing, or playing music, as a way to channel your emotions.

Seek solitude and relaxation: Find a quiet space to relax and calm your mind. Engage in activities like meditation, progressive muscle relaxation, or visualization techniques.

Set realistic expectations: Understand that not everything will go your way. Accept that you can't control everything, and focus on what you can change.

Practice forgiveness: Letting go of grudges and forgiving others (and yourself) can help release built-up anger and promote emotional healing.

Addressing the Ups and Downs of Your Emotions

Maybe you can accept that your emotions will get the better of you at times. You may feel anxious, irritated, or even angry for what seems like no reason. If these emotional swings happen too often and with regularity, and interfere with your quality of life, don't just blame it all on your perimenopause. Other problems — real relationship issues, family complications, or medical problems — may cause (or, at least, contribute to) these bouts of emotional upheaval.

Seeking counseling

Counseling — specifically, anger management therapy, whether in a group setting or in a one-on-one therapy session — can help you find skills to cope with, prevent, and redirect anger and rage. Sometimes, you may benefit from couples or family therapy, as well, if family or relationship issues seem to be adding to your overall emotional upheaval during perimenopause.

If you can locate a good counselor or therapist, they can help you sort out whether your symptoms are related to hormonal changes accompanying midlife or are truly mental health issues that just happened to coincide with your major life transition.

You can find a therapist by asking your primary care physician or your gynecologist for a referral; if you feel comfortable, ask your friends for the name of a therapist that they have had success with; there are also many online therapists (BetterHelp.com, Onlinetherapy.com). It's important to find someone who is a fit, and someone you feel comfortable talking to.

Cognitive behavioral therapy (CBT) is a type of psychotherapy that can show you how to modify emotions, behaviors, and thoughts that are dysfunctional to your life, as well as how to develop personal coping strategies. CBT helps you find practical ways of managing your problems and focuses on the links between physical symptoms and behavior.

Self-calming with yoga and relaxation

You can use a variety of relaxation techniques and paced breathing to calm down your body's physical and emotional reactions. Yoga, meditation, and rhythmic breathing all provide you with self-calming skills that you can use to handle your fluctuating emotions. A regular exercise routine can help boost your body image and banish negative thoughts that lead to irritation and anger.

Checking out anger management

Anger management is a psychotherapy program for the prevention and control of anger. It teaches how to deploy anger successfully. Because anger is often the result of frustration or a feeling of being blocked, this particular type of therapy helps to identify anger issues, teaching how to control anger to prevent feeling out of control. The goal is to keep your anger from impacting your life and relationships.

Boosting endorphins by exercising

The links between depression, anxiety, and exercise aren't entirely clear. But regular exercise can help relieve depression and anxiety in a number of ways. Exercise:

>> Helps release something called *endorphins,* natural cannabis-like brain chemicals that can help enhance your sense of well-being

>> Can help you get away from the irritability, anxiety, and depression that come from a cycle of negative thought

>> Is a positive coping strategy because it's healthy, can be sociable, and can help you gain confidence as you meet your exercise goals and challenges

REMEMBER

Small amounts of physical activity — as little as 10 to 15 minutes at a time — can make a difference; setting reasonable and realistic goals can help you stick to a program. Exercise can help ease your symptoms of depression and anxiety, but it's not a substitute for therapy or medication if symptoms don't seem to be relieved with regular physical activity.

Making time for mindfulness

Mindfulness means maintaining a moment-to-moment awareness of your thoughts, feelings, bodily sensations, and surrounding environment through a gentle, nurturing lens. When you practice mindfulness, your thoughts tune into what you're sensing now, instead of rehashing the past or imagining the future. Mindfulness programs and apps are aimed at stress reduction and can help you avoid destructive automatic habits and responses by figuring out how to observe your thoughts in the moment. Mindfulness is the basic human ability to be fully present, aware of where you are and what you're doing, and to avoid becoming overly reactive to what's going on around you.

Here are some mindfulness websites to check out:

>> **Mindful** (www.mindful.org): A website meant to facilitate engaging with your life and your moments through the ongoing cultivation of mindfulness.

>> **PsychCentral** (www.psychcentral.com): A website with information on many different mental health conditions: ADHD, anxiety, bipolar disorder, depression and PTSD. It discusses various wellness topics and offers support.

>> **Calm** (www.calm.com): An app to help improve sleep quality, reduce stress and anxiety, improve focus, and concentrate on self-improvement.

>> **Headspace** (www.headspace.com): An app that helps with mindfulness, meditation, and self-care.

Prioritizing sleep

Poor sleep is more than just an annoyance. It's linked to many chronic health problems, including heart disease, kidney disease, high blood pressure, stroke, and depression. Not getting enough sleep drains your mental abilities and puts your physical health at risk. It causes increased stress levels and, in turn, increased anxiety levels. Having good *sleep hygiene* — going to bed at the same time every night; keeping the room cool; limiting food, alcohol, and caffeine close to bedtime; and having a relaxing bedtime ritual — can all help improve the quantity and quality of your sleep. (See Chapter 11 for more about sleep changes during perimenopause.) Mental and emotional health (as well as physical health) take a nosedive when you don't make sleep a priority.

Seeking out supplements

Doctors don't have definitive evidence that supplementing certain vitamins can have a direct effect on improving mental and emotional health. Here's a breakdown of the connections between vitamins and mental health:

» **Vitamin B-12 and other B vitamins:** These seem to have some effect on depressed mood because a deficiency of these vitamins can worsen depression.

» **Vitamin D:** Deficiency of this vitamin can cause depressive symptoms Research suggests that vitamin D deficiency is linked to a higher risk of depression.

» **Multivitamin:** If you're suffering from severe anxiety or depression, you may be less likely to take care of yourself, including eating a healthy and varied diet; if you find yourself not eating a balanced diet, take a daily multivitamin designed for midlife women.

   A multivitamin may have enough of the required and recommended doses of vitamins, but taking a multivitamin doesn't provide treatment for any particular mental health condition.

Perimenopause seems to have come around at a time in your life designed for maximum stress: You may be dealing with children in their teens or older; parents who may be ill and need caretaking; a relationship that you may have to take a good hard look at; and jobs that may be asking more of you. Who wouldn't get angry, anxious, or depressed sometimes?

If those feelings are persistent, growing, or disturbing, see a doctor for a full mental health evaluation. Armed with this chapter, you know what to ask your doctor and to advocate for a checkup, not just for your physical health, but for that all-important probe into the inner workings of your mind.

Using medication to stabilize your moods

You may want to consider several categories of medications if alternatives and home remedies (which I talk about in the preceding sections), and all the exercise in the world (covered in the section "Boosting endorphins by exercising," earlier in this chapter) doesn't seem to help your moods while you make the (sometimes many years) long menopausal transition.

Medications, including those you can take to create hormonal balance (some types of hormonal birth control or hormone therapy) and those that work directly on the release and availability of neurotransmitters such as serotonin and dopamine, may provide the stability that you're sorely missing in the perimenopausal transition. Initiate this discussion with your doctor if they're unaware of these changes or they don't ask about them.

You and your doctor may decide to try one medication, and then add another if you're not getting the relief that you need. Or you can try one, and then switch to another if it's not having the effect you want. You may even try several medications in different categories until something clicks.

What if you had a medication that helps relieve hot flashes and, at the very same time, increases the neurotransmitters that treat depression and anxiety? Well, there are several classes of medication that can do this. Selective serotonin reuptake inhibitors (SSRIs) and serotonin-norepinephrine reuptake inhibitors (SNRIs) are both used to treat hot flashes along with depression and anxiety. Some common SSRIs and SNRIs include:

>> **Venlafaxine (Effexor):** Increases not only serotonin levels but also other neurotransmitters (dopamine and norepinephrine). At the lower doses it mostly has its effect on serotonin.

>> **Paroxetine (Paxil):** Increases the levels of serotonin in the brain.

>> **Duloxetine (Cymbalta):** Increases the amount of serotonin in the brain, along with increasing the levels of norepinephrine.

>> **Escitalopram (Lexapro):** Available in both a tablet and a liquid, it also works by increasing the amount of serotonin in the brain.

>> **Fluoxetine (Prozac):** Increases the serotonin levels in the brain as well.

The antidepressant bupropion (Wellbutrin) works by increasing norepinephrine and dopamine in the brain and may help treat perimenopausal anxiety and depression with fewer sexual side effects than SSRIs have.

Some women who take SSRIs report *low libido,* a decrease in sexual interest. You and your doctor must do a delicate balancing act to treat one set of symptoms by taking medications that themselves cause another set of symptoms that you may find unacceptable. Especially at midlife, you already have so many other sexual changes taking place (see Chapter 7 for a discussion of what perimenopause can do to your sex life).

Although Chapter 6 reviews whether you want to start or continue certain types of hormonal therapy during perimenopause, this section looks specifically at whether hormones can treat the perimenopausal emotional and mental health conditions of depression, anxiety, and irritability. After all, if the wide swings of naturally produced hormones in your midlife body (coming from your midlife ovaries) seem to be causing these emotional changes, why not just take hormones as a mood stabilizer? Sometimes, that's not a bad idea.

But remember that hormones aren't a treatment for the diagnosis of depression or anxiety. No one knows exactly how declining hormone levels may cause depression, but estrogen and serotonin levels are somehow linked.

By stabilizing estrogen and progesterone, you may experience an increase in serotonin levels, which in turn provides relief for anxiety and depression. Only a serious discussion with a medical professional can help you decide whether to use hormone therapy as a safe addition to an overall treatment plan for your mental health.

Chapter **10**

Looking After You: Practicing Self-Care

This book has been written to specifically address the concerns of women who are going through their perimenopausal years: the years at the end of fertility and reproduction, and at the beginning of menopause. With so many (often unanticipated) changes taking place in your body, your mind, and your relationships, you may have difficulty maintaining a strong sense of self.

However, perimenopause provides a perfect time to look at your relationship with yourself, work on resilience and self-improvement, and look forward to the rest of your life.

In this chapter, you can read about methods of shifting away from self-criticism, to discover and connect with your strengths and self-value, and to focus on self-care, with advice on taking good care of you. Many ideas in this chapter are inspired by *Resilience For Dummies*, by Eva M. Selhub, M.D. (Wiley).

Practicing Resilience

What does it mean to be resilient? People who possess this quality take responsibility for their actions and attitudes. As a woman in perimenopause, this is particularly powerful. Be forward thinking, working on yourself continuously and looking to improve yourself and your life. Because resilient people possess a positive self-image, they feel capable of moving in the direction of their goals, undeterred by moments of failure and doubt.

By being resilient, you can more confidently move through your perimenopausal journey toward menopause. Also, resilient people tend to have healthy relationships and maintain a strong sense of accomplishment, so even if some of the changes your body is going through may lower your confidence, if you are resilient, you can quiet the voices of doubt and move on.

Resilience doesn't rely on positive outcomes or beneficial circumstances: Resilient people have a positive self-belief and self-image, no matter what's happening in or around them. Here are two clear ways to stay resilient through perimenopause:

>> Remember past successes, such as the time you single-handedly planned a charity event or gave a speech in front of a room full of colleagues. Continue to celebrate those successes and remember how good you felt.

>> View setbacks as opportunities, like when you found yourself a little lost and ended up able to explore a new city on your own.

REMEMBER

You may find staying resilient more difficult in midlife because so many aspects of your body and your life are changing, and you may find your sense of self-worth and value affected by a feeling that you have no control over many of these changes. Your sense of your own capabilities may take a hit when your body and/or your brain seem to be failing you.

Most resilient people share several traits that reflect a positive self-image, which invariably enables them to get through hardship and major life changes.

Practice these actions to help build your resilience:

>> **Avoid being affected by others' opinions.** Don't worry about what the media thinks of menopausal women, and never let yourself feel devalued because of age.

>> **Recognize your uniqueness.** Understand what makes you unique and stay true to those things. Show and embrace your true self.

>> **Take pride in achievements.** Although you always want to have new goals in your sights, take time to acknowledge past achievements, too — even if it's just not biting someone's head off on a bad day.

» **Maintain a growth mindset.** Hold on to your desire to be better. Don't see this time in life as the end of your sense of adventure or your ability to achieve new things.

» **Show self-compassion.** Be kind to yourself, rather than constantly critical.

» **Embrace mistakes.** If brain fog leads you to make a mistake, don't look at the situation as a huge setback; think of it as an opportunity to really evaluate your problem-solving skills.

» **Self-reflect.** Make time in your life to think about your emotions and feelings and try to understand them. Can you make positive changes to your situation?

» **Practice gratitude.** If you really want to feel successful, count your blessings and feel gratitude. While you go through this stage in your life, think about all the things you have already accomplished.

Keeping a Positive Attitude

When you see the possibilities in a difficult situation (such as letting the anger you may feel at your spouse get the better of you and lashing out) and believe in your own worth, you can better recover from missteps or mistakes, as well as keep your determination when you meet setbacks. Try to keep yourself in this frame of mind while you experience the ups and downs of perimenopause:

» **Persevere.** Avoid viewing mistakes and setbacks as failures, and try to see opportunities all around you. Your self-belief gives you the courage and drive to persist and keep going.

» **Stay open.** Don't worry about being judged or making mistakes; you can be open, curious, and receptive to what life has to offer you. Accept advice and guidance as helpful and constructive, rather than critical. Trust friends who have gone through something similar to guide you through the experience.

» **Believe in the possible.** Believe in yourself and your ability to find solutions and achieve a desired outcome.

Know that other people believe in you, as well. Others want to accompany you on your life journey.

» **Take care.** Value yourself, and always take the necessary time for self-care. If you nurture yourself physically and emotionally, you can better handle the unexpected and unpredictable aspects of perimenopause. Others may need you, but you cannot care for others if you don't care for yourself.

Maintaining Healthy Boundaries

Know when to give to others and when to focus on taking care of yourself. Make your values and priorities known, and express your needs clearly. Women are often reluctant to say no when asked to help or to take on additional work. Maintaining healthy boundaries is essential for your well-being and relationships.

Here are some ways to establish and maintain healthy boundaries:

>> **Self-awareness:** Reflect on what makes you comfortable and uncomfortable in various situations. Start by understanding your needs, values, and limits. This self-awareness will guide you in setting appropriate boundaries.

>> **Communication:** Effective communication is the key to establishing and maintaining boundaries. Clearly and assertively express your boundaries to others. Practice being honest and direct while considering their feelings.

>> **Focus on self-care:** Taking care of your physical, emotional, and mental well-being allows you to establish boundaries from a place of strength and self-respect.

>> **Learn to say no:** Realize that you have the right to decline requests, invitations, or demands. Saying no when necessary is a crucial part of boundary-setting.

>> **Evaluate your relationships:** Try to determine whether your relationships are healthy and supportive of your boundaries. Unhealthy relationships violate your boundaries, and you should consider whether to terminate them.

>> **Respect others' boundaries:** Just as you expect others to respect your boundaries, honor the boundaries set by others. This promotes healthy interactions.

You may find maintaining these boundaries especially difficult in perimenopause because you're in a time in your life where relationships and responsibilities around you are changing. It's normal to encounter resistance from others when you first establish boundaries, especially if you have not been a boundary-setter in the past. Staying consistent and prioritizing your well-being will ultimately lead to more balanced relationships and a greater sense of self-worth and self-respect.

Taking care of aging parents, raising children that are growing more independent, and changes in your professional and personal relationships are all happening at a time when you also have physical and emotional changes suddenly upon you. Maintaining healthy boundaries and practicing self-care are essential at this time.

TIP

Staying informed and prepared for many of these changes (such as reading this book and surrounding yourself with supportive people) can help you feel capable of overcoming challenges and balancing your care for others with your self-care.

Practicing Self-Awareness

To recognize your value, you need to become truly self-aware; to be aware of what you're feeling at any particular moment, without judgment or evaluation. When you're self-aware, you can consciously choose in which direction you want to go.

Most people can be their own harshest critics:

>> If you're wracked with self-doubt, how do you respond to criticism?

>> If you don't believe in your abilities to live your life by yourself, how might you leave an unhealthy relationship?

>> Do you congratulate yourself when you succeed, and take good care of yourself, even if the outcome wasn't what you expected or wanted?

To move through this sometimes difficult perimenopausal transition, accept yourself as you are, acknowledge a desire for growth, and make yourself accountable for your actions while still valuing yourself.

When you start paying attention to your behavior, thoughts, feelings, and beliefs, you can begin to notice any negative thoughts: how often you

>> Put yourself down

>> Look for validation

>> Compare yourself to others

>> Engage in self-defeating thoughts or behaviors

Self-awareness and self-examination are an ongoing process. Whatever you notice tells you more about yourself and helps you discover where the negative thoughts and beliefs may originate.

REMEMBER

When you accumulate observations for self-examination, also note the times when you feel confident and successful. Try to make a conscious choice to feel positive about yourself more often than not. Choose not to empower negative thoughts and instead to focus on your value.

Keeping Inventory of Yourself

Identify your strengths, abilities, and qualities that are unique to you. Make sure that you remain mindful of yourself and all that you can do:

» **Take an inventory.** Create an ongoing inventory of your qualities, competencies, and accomplishments.

» **Pause to reflect.** When you feel good about something you do, take a moment to reflect on your qualities or abilities that enabled you to accomplish this feat. Maybe you were able to complete a strenuous hike because you trained for weeks.

» **Count everything.** Keep track of all your successful qualities if you managed to

   • Always get to work on time (qualities of being responsible and punctual)

   • Successfully pull off planning a surprise party (qualities of discreteness and resourcefulness)

   • Resolve conflict between friends (empathetic and an effective communicator)

   Everything counts!

» **Review your positive qualities.** Regularly read over your list, and remind yourself of your positive qualities and the ways that you're valuable and valued.

» **Note areas of your life where you want to grow and improve.** Perimenopause, as a transitional period, provides the perfect time to look for any weaknesses that you may have in how you approach life, as well as noting and evaluating setbacks and situations where your efforts weren't successful.

Taking Care of You

You can nurture your body to stay strong and vibrant while you move through your perimenopausal years and into menopause. You have control over

» **Your exercise routine:** Chapter 14 dives into staying (or becoming) physically fit during perimenopause.

» **Healthy nutrition:** You can read all about eating healthy during perimenopause in Chapter 13.

>> **A good, restorative sleep regimen:** Chapter 11 deals with what perimenopause does to your sleep routine and what you can do to counteract those changes.

>> **Stress-relief and meditation:** Make sure to have a "go-to" when stress starts to creep up: Exercise, mindfulness apps, a social circle, a trusted therapist can all be sources of stress relief.

When you feel strong and healthy physically, you have more energy, and that energy supports your mental attitude and ability to handle challenges. Don't let go of positive self-care behaviors when you're under stress from many simultaneous changes in your life as well as changes in your relationship with work.

Instead of looking outward for people, places, and things to complete you, focus on people, places, and things that can support you so that you can be your best. Figure out how to have a deep connection with yourself and to do what you can to support yourself so that you can thrive.

Keep this list in mind for taking good care of you:

>> Nourish yourself with nutrient-rich food (see Chapter 13).

>> Exercise and stay active (flip to Chapter 14).

>> Connect with support: friends, family, social networks, your physician or therapist.

>> Quiet your mind and take some time to rest.

>> Have fun!

>> Appreciate all that you have and all that you are (techniques for which I discuss in the preceding section).

Cultivating calm amidst the storm

During perimenopause, you may feel increased levels of stress and anxiety on a regular basis. To counteract the effects of added stress, incorporate stress-reduction techniques into your daily routine to help alleviate anxiety, improve focus, and enhance overall well-being:

>> Deep breathing exercises

>> Meditation (see the following section)

>> Mindfulness practices

By dedicating time to these practices, you not only fortify your mental and emotional health, but also cultivate a sense of calm that can greatly benefit ease your path through major life transitions.

Letting love in

While you travel through your midlife years and move from perimenopause into menopause, set your intentions on a path to loving yourself. Believe in your own ability to create and to have joy, ease, comfort, and love. Do what you need to do to feel alive, vibrant, and healthy. When you feel good, you radiate goodness, and you attract more of the same.

You don't have to wait for other people to give you love to have it. You can do it yourself by opening your heart to love itself and by acting. You can allow love in by

>> Practicing gratitude and appreciation

>> Being vulnerable and asking for help from your support network, whether they are family, friends, neighbors, colleagues, or medical professionals

>> Intentionally nurturing yourself through your self-care practices (including nutrition, sleep, exercise, and stress reduction)

>> Spending time in nature and feeling a sense of connection and awe

>> Allowing yourself to feel your feelings, whether positive or negative, and seeing all of yourself as valuable

Opening your heart through meditation

If you've never meditated, or are only somewhat familiar with the practice, it can be a little intimidating — perhaps even feel a bit strange — at the start. There's really no right or wrong way to meditate. If you choose to try a guided mediation, you can do so

>> In a group, such as at an organized meditation retreat or class

>> With a meditation teacher, who can be found through a community or religious center

>> Through an app that you can use to find guided meditation at various lengths and for many purposes

>> On guided meditation YouTube channels

>> By reading books like *Wherever You Go There You Are* by Jon Kabat-Zinn and *The Power of Now* by Eckhart Tolle

Follow these steps to try a meditation exercise:

1. **Find a comfortable position.**

   Make it somewhere quiet where no one will disturb you.

2. **Close your eyes and bring your awareness to the center of your chest.**

   This area is known as the *heart center*.

3. **Gently breathe into and out of the heart center, counting 1-2-3 while you breathe in and 1-2-3-4-5-6 while you breathe out.**

4. **While you breathe in and out, observe any sensations or feelings that you're experiencing in your chest.**

   Does your chest feel open, closed, relaxed, tight, heavy, or light?

5. **Observe what emotions you feel.**

   Observe without judgment. Don't label whatever you feel as right or wrong.

6. **Be aware that you're observing energy in your heart and noticing what it feels like.**

7. **Imagine your breath starting to move the energy in your chest, like a curtain that moves with the breeze.**

   It's effortless. Just let it move in and out with your breath.

8. **While you breathe in, imagine that you're breathing in unlimited love and infinite intelligence from the universe into your heart.**

9. **When you exhale, imagine that you're simply letting go of everything else.**

   Breathe in unlimited love and infinite intelligence, exhaling and letting go of everything else.

10. **Continue to breathe in and out.**

    With every breath, imagine that your heart fills with unlimited love and infinite intelligence until it's so full that this love and intelligence begin to overflow.

11. **Observe that there's no separation between your heart and the heart of the entire universe.**

    Because you're connected by unlimited love and infinite intelligence.

12. Say to yourself, "Our hearts are one heart."

13. Picture your heart connecting with other hearts.

14. Visualize unlimited love and infinite intelligence flowing freely between the hearts.

15. Repeat the phrase, "Our hearts are one heart."

Stay in this state as long as you want.

16. When you're ready, give thanks for the fullness of your heart and the fullness of your being.

After a meditation session is over, most people will feel a sense of relaxation. You may feel a decrease in anxiety and stress. Sometimes, meditation can bring about a sense of mental clarity and focus, or a feeling of calm. You may feel a sense of heightened awareness and a reduced perception of pain. Not every meditation session will result in all of these feelings. The effects of meditation can be subtle and cumulative; they may become more pronounced with regular practice over time.

Taking Care of Yourself in the Workplace

Extend your self-care practices to the workplace. While women transition through perimenopause, the workplace can sometimes feel like uncharted territory. However, with the right support, it can become a space of empowerment and understanding.

In the following sections, I explore various strategies and initiatives that employers can implement to provide crucial support during this transformative phase.

Don't think that the workplace needs to be a source of additional stress or discomfort. Through a combination of flexible arrangements, thoughtful environmental adjustments, open communication, and stress-reduction techniques, you can find a balance that allows you to thrive professionally while honoring the changes taking place within you.

Flexible work arrangements: Finding balance amidst change

One of the most effective ways employers can support women navigating perimenopause is by offering flexible work arrangements. This flexibility can be a game-changer for those grappling with disrupted sleep patterns and persistent fatigue. By working closely with your manager, you can discuss the possibility of adjusting your working hours. This change might entail starting later in the day or having the option to work from home, or even adopting a hybrid model that blends office and remote work.

TIP

These accommodations can be instrumental in helping you strike a balance between your professional responsibilities and the physical challenges posed by perimenopause.

Temperature control: Creating comfortable work environments

Hot flashes, the hallmark of perimenopause, can be not only physically uncomfortable, but also emotionally challenging in a professional setting. To alleviate this discomfort, you have some options:

>> **Climate control:** Consider working in areas that have effective temperature control. If possible, adjust the air conditioning settings or use fans to regulate the environment.

>> **Perimenopause-friendly dress code:** Advocate for a relaxing dress code if you possibly can opt for cooler fabrics, such as linen, and looser clothing that allows for better air circulation. Body temperature fluctuations can be more bearable if you have layers of clothing that you can adjust depending on the temperature of the office and of your body.

TIP

If your job requires a uniform, don't hesitate to inquire about adjustments that can make it more breathable and comfortable.

Establishing open communication channels

Your workplace needs to establish open lines of communication between employees and supervisors, as well as with the HR department, to create a supportive work environment. This openness allows for candid discussions about your needs and potential accommodations that your employer and coworkers can make to assist you during this transitional phase.

When everyone is informed and receptive, it paves the way for a collaborative approach to navigating perimenopause in the workplace. Whether you need scheduling adjustments, workspace modifications, or other considerations, open communication ensures that your work community understands and addresses your unique needs.

Chapter **11**

The Elusive Full Night of Sleep

You've probably had the experience of lying awake in bed, staring at the ceiling, and willing yourself to just go to sleep. Maybe you're trying to first fall asleep (and know you have an important meeting in the morning). Maybe you randomly wake up in the middle of the night, only to stare at the ceiling, listen to your heart beating, or check the clock ticking ever-so-slowly. Or maybe you wake up just a few hours before you have to, and you find yourself asking, "Is it even worth it to go back to sleep?"

Whichever scenario you find yourself in, losing sleep disrupts the rest of your day; in your waking hours, you want to be sharp, have focus, and stay awake for a work meeting, a movie, or your kid's soccer game. Losing sleep pretty much makes you feel tired all the time, and when you feel tired all the time, your physical and mental health suffer.

The effects of poor sleep extend beyond tiredness and poor performance. Long-term sleep disruptions can alter brain chemistry, which can lead to anxiety, depression, and other mental health disorders.

In this chapter, you can examine how changes in perimenopause impact your sleep and consider the science of falling asleep, staying asleep, sleep hygiene, and how you may be sabotaging your own sleep plan.

Understanding Sleep during Perimenopause

One of the most common complaints that women have during this time of perimenopause is about their seemingly sudden inability to get a good night's sleep. Many perimenopausal women experience disrupted sleep patterns that can last through to menopause.

Losing sleep is very much something to lose sleep over. Together with other symptoms that you may experience (which I talk about through Parts 2 and 3 of this book), sleepless nights make everything feel that much harder.

If you wake up tired and feel fatigued throughout the day since entering this stage of midlife called perimenopause, your body probably isn't spending enough time in the deep stages of sleep at night.

Whether you experience these sleep changes because of fluctuating hormones, anxiety, temperature dysregulation, or any number of other suddenly appearing and unexpected perimenopausal symptoms, you have many ways to restore that good quality sleep. Your bed should be a place for the only two things that should happen there: great sleep and great sex.

Identifying How Hormones Affect Sleep

Perhaps you remember times in your younger life when you saw your bed as a respite. You just needed a few plush pillows and a fleece blanket, and you could curl up for the night — out cold. Those days likely live on only in memory. Whether you have trouble falling asleep, staying asleep, or anything in between, that bed can represent a battleground. You can't seem to get comfortable on those plush pillows, and you have to throw that fleece blanket on and off yourself more times than you care to count. What makes sleep so elusive in perimenopause?

Well, sleep — especially good sleep — is all about the routine; your body thrives on a regular and consistent sleep-wake cycle. Perimenopause disrupts that routine, introducing all kinds of transitions, changes, and fluctuations.

Hormonal fluctuations can affect quality and length of sleep in up to half of women undergoing the perimenopausal transition. Levels of estrogen and progesterone, the two main hormones made by the ovaries, start to decline at midlife, and your hormone levels will fluctuate for years during perimenopause. These fluctuations cause a host of symptoms, many of which contribute to poor sleep.

Hormonal fluctuations can affect sleep in a number of ways:

>> **Body temperature regulation:** Especially changes in estrogen levels can cause an inability for your body to regulate its own temperature. The thermostat of your body just doesn't work. When your body can't regulate its own temperature, you may experience hot flashes during the day and night sweats when you try to sleep.

These swings in the thermometer can certainly interrupt a good night of sleep because you wake up covered in sweat, and you have to throw off the covers or even change your clothing to re-regulate your body's temperature.

>> **GABA production:** The perimenopausal decrease in *progesterone* (a hormone that has a calming, sedative effect) often makes falling asleep more difficult. Progesterone promotes sleep by stimulating the brain to produce a chemical (also known as a *neurotransmitter*) called gamma-amino-butyric acid (GABA). GABA promotes a sleep-inducing or hypnotic effect that can help trigger normal sleep cycles.

>> **Melatonin production:** A hormone produced by the brain in response to darkness, *melatonin* plays a part in the sleep-wake cycle. Declining levels of estrogen, and aging in general, cause a decrease in the production of melatonin by the brain. Decreasing levels can impact the consistency of these cycles, making it more difficult to fall asleep and stay asleep.

>> **Other hormone-related symptoms:** Symptoms that occur because of hormonal fluctuation at midlife — such as urinary frequency, anxiety, stress, poor concentration, and mood swings — can also lead to interrupted sleep. Getting up at night to use the bathroom, or staying awake while you constantly think about the stressors of the day, can also contribute to that feeling in the morning that you just can't seem to get a restorative night of sleep.

Hot flashes

Daytime *hot flashes*, a feeling of heat rushing over your body several (or many) times a day, commonly occur during perimenopause and menopause. When this sensation happens at night, it is referred to it as *night sweats*, when you wake up flushed and covered in perspiration. Sometimes, this sweat can saturate your clothing and bedsheets.

Although infections, thyroid conditions, and certain medications can cause hot flashes and night sweats, these symptoms often happen because of the fluctuating hormone levels of perimenopause. You may not realize that a night sweat woke you; only after you wake up and notice your soaked pajamas do you realize that the sweating woke you. And now, you just can't fall back asleep — even after you change your clothes.

Insomnia

Insomnia, the inability to fall asleep or stay asleep, can happen at any age. But it seems to more commonly occur while you age. Insomnia can sap not only your daytime energy level and mood, but also take a toll on your health, work performance, and quality of life:

>> **Short-term:** If you experience a traumatic or stressful event, it may cause short-term insomnia, which can last from a few days to a few weeks; you just can't shut down thoughts about this event at the end of the day.

>> **Long-term:** If you experience long-term insomnia, lasting a few months or longer, seek medical help to determine a cause and treatment before this chronic condition has permanent effects on your long-term health.

Restless leg syndrome

Restless leg syndrome causes an uncontrollable urge to move your legs, usually at night, because of an uncomfortable sensation. Moving them seems to temporarily ease that unpleasant sensation. It can disrupt sleep and interfere with your daily activities. The sensation typically begins after you sit or lie down for an extended period of time, and you can relieve it by stretching, movement, or jiggling your legs. Sometimes, women feel this sensation as a numbness or throbbing that's difficult to explain.

The cause for this condition is unknown, although your doctor may do blood work to check for iron deficiency or diabetes.

Your doctor can choose from several medications to treat this condition after you have an exam and evaluation. Keep in mind that the choice of medication and dosage should be determined by a healthcare professional based on your specific situation.

Here are some common medications used to treat RLS:

Dopaminergic medications

Dopaminergic agents can be effective in alleviating the symptoms of RLS because they can help regulate dopamine levels in the brain.

Here are some dopaminergic agents your doctor may prescribe:

>> **Pramipexole (Mirapex):** This medication stimulates dopamine receptors in the brain and is commonly used to treat RLS. It is available in both immediate-release and extended-release forms.

>> **Ropinirole (Requip):** Like pramipexole, ropinirole is a dopamine agonist. It can also be prescribed for RLS.

>> **Rotigotine (Neupro):** This is a dopamine agonist delivered via a transdermal patch.

Alpha-2-delta ligands

Alpha-2-delta ligands are drugs that play a role in transmitting pain signals in the central nervous system.

Here are some medications in this category:

>> **Gabapentin enacarbil (Horizant):** This medication is structurally related to gabapentin and is specifically approved for treating moderate to severe RLS.

>> **Pregabalin (Lyrica):** Although primarily used to treat neuropathic pain and epilepsy, pregabalin can also be effective in managing RLS symptoms.

Iron supplements

Your doctor may prescribe iron supplements, because iron deficiency is identified as a contributing factor to RLS.

Anticonvulsants

A medication called carbamazepine (Tegretol) is sometimes used for its anticonvulsant properties in the treatment of RLS.

Sleep apnea

Doctors diagnose more than 200,000 new cases of sleep apnea in the U.S. every year. *Sleep apnea,* a potentially serious sleep disorder, occurs when your breathing repeatedly stops and starts throughout the night, causing sleep disruptions and daytime fatigue. Symptoms include loud snoring, nighttime restlessness, and feeling fatigued even after a full night of sleep.

Diagnosis of sleep apnea requires a medical evaluation. Your doctor takes a detailed sleep and lifestyle history, and they often order a sleep study. A *sleep study*, which you can sometimes do at home, but which occurs more often in a sleep laboratory, monitors your heart rate, lung activity, and brain activity for one or more nights. You also may need to make a visit to a *cardiologist* (heart specialist) and/or an ear-nose and throat specialist, checking for all possible reasons for obstruction.

Treatment for sleep apnea often consists of

>> **Self-care:** Such as increasing exercise, quitting smoking, and losing weight.

>> **CPAP:** Your healthcare provider might prescribe a continuous positive airway pressure (CPAP) device to assist your nighttime breathing. These devices deliver air pressure through a mask on your nose and/or mouth while you sleep.

> You can find all different types of masks and various airway pressure devices; figure out the one that works best for you.

>> **Surgery:** Your healthcare provider and you may consider surgery an option, usually only when all other treatments have failed. A surgeon can remove tissue from the top of your throat and the rear of your mouth, or you can potentially have surgery to reposition your jaw.

TIP

I outline the different types of sleep apnea in the following sections.

Obstructive sleep apnea (OSA)

Obstructive sleep apnea (OSA) is the most common form of sleep apnea. It occurs when throat muscles relax and block the flow of air into the lungs during sleep. When these muscles relax, the airway narrows while you breathe in. Because you can't get enough air into your lungs, you consequently don't get enough oxygen. The brain senses this lack of oxygen and briefly wakes you up so that you can reposition and reopen the airway.

This pattern generally repeats itself somewhere between 5 and 30 times each hour, which makes it hard or impossible to reach the deep restful phase of sleep.

Some well-known risk factors for the obstructive form of sleep apnea include

>> **Excess weight:** Obesity greatly increases the risk of OSA. Fat deposits around the neck and upper airway can obstruct breathing.

>> **Thicker neck circumference:** People who have thicker necks tend to have narrower airways.

>> **An inherited narrow airway:** Sleep apnea may run in families; you may have inherited a narrow airway or throat.

- >> **Tonsilitis:** Tonsils can be enlarged or swollen and block the airway.

- >> **Age:** Sleep apnea occurs significantly more in older adults.

- >> **Use of alcohol, sedatives, and tranquilizers:** All of these substances relax the muscles in the throat, which can cause or worsen sleep apnea.

- >> **Nasal congestion:** If you have trouble breathing through your nose (from allergies or anatomy).

- >> **Certain medical conditions:** If you have type 2 diabetes, high blood pressure, or congestive heart failure.

Complex sleep apnea

Complex sleep apnea is also known as *treatment-emergent sleep apnea.* It happens when a patient who's receiving treatment for obstructive sleep apnea (OSA; discussed in the preceding section) converts to central sleep apnea (CSA; see the following section) during treatment for sleep apnea.

Central sleep apnea

Central sleep apnea (CSA) involves a problem with brain signaling. The brain doesn't send the proper stimulation to the muscles that control breathing. Because your brain doesn't tell your body to breathe while you sleep, you awaken with shortness of breath several times per night, creating difficulty staying asleep. The following factors can increase the risk of developing central sleep apnea:

- >> Use of narcotic pain medications

- >> History of stroke or congestive heart failure

- >> Age (middle-aged or older)

Searching for the Holy Grail: More (and Better) Sleep

The accumulation of nights, weeks, or even months of poor sleep can ultimately have a detrimental effect on your body and your quality of life. Lack of sleep leads to inflammation and weight gain, poor daytime performance and a multitude of health problems. The goal of better sleep is one worth pursuing during your perimenopausal transition. Go for it!

Like all issues you may encounter during perimenopause, no one single solution can guarantee you better sleep. If you put a good night of sleep high on your list of goals during this midlife transition (and you really should!), you may need to make a combination of commitments to achieve it. You'll find the effort you need to put in so worth it when you start feeling rested in the morning and able to function clearly throughout your day.

The following sections offer some ways in which you can improve your chances of getting consistent nights of deep, healthy sleep.

Improving sleep hygiene

Although you probably want to wash up before getting into bed for the night, the term *sleep hygiene* actually refers to the habits and practices that can help you sleep well on a regular basis. Good sleep habits can improve both the length of time you sleep and how deep you sleep, and poor sleep hygiene can have exactly the opposite effect.

Think of how you would put a baby to sleep. You can use many of the steps on a new-mother checklist for getting a baby to fall asleep for yourself, particularly in perimenopause.

Here's a list to keep in mind when you want to find that elusive night's slumber:

>> Be consistent. Plan to go to sleep at the same time every night.

>> Make your bedroom quiet, dark, relaxing, and a comfortable temperature.

>> Remove electronic devices, such as televisions, computers, tablets, and smart phones from the bedroom.

>> Create a relaxing bedtime routine to get your mind and body ready for sleep. You can read (using low reading lights), take a hot bath, use a meditation app, or practice deep breathing.

>> Use earplugs, a sleep mask, and/or a white noise machine to keep things dark, quiet, and without distractions.

>> Skip caffeinated beverages within six hours of bedtime.

>> Avoid alcohol for at least three hours prior to bedtime.

>> Avoid eating big meals close to bedtime, especially spicy foods.

>> Try not to nap during the day. If you must nap, do so early in the day, not close to bedtime.

>> Spend time during the day in the sun (wearing sunscreen), but avoid bright lights close to bedtime.

>> Use your bed for only either sleep or sex.

>> Try to get 20 minutes of brisk exercise daily.

TIP

Aim for at least seven or eight hours of uninterrupted sleep per night. If you follow the advice in the preceding list and still can't fall asleep or stay asleep, you may need to talk to your medical provider to get a complete evaluation and hopefully come up with some good solutions for your sleep woes.

Using supplements as sleep aids

Some studies have shown that certain supplements can help you fall and stay asleep. But consult your healthcare provider before you start any supplement because you may have specific medical reasons that you shouldn't take them.

Melatonin

Melatonin is a hormone produced by the body that signals to the brain that it's time to go to sleep. Melatonin supplements have become popular, especially for situations in which the sleep-wake cycle gets disrupted, such as during travel (and jet lag). Melatonin appears to reduce the amount of time it takes to fall asleep. Studies have observed that melatonin in doses of 3 to 10 milligrams (mg) may have a positive effect on sleep, and these doses appear to be safe for adults in the short term. (Avoid gummies that have added sugar, which can counteract restfulness.)

Valerian root

For centuries, *valerian root* has been used to treat anxiety, depression, and insomnia. Not many reliable studies have been conducted, and some women find they experience the opposite effect — this herb causes them to stay awake. However, a small study found that taking 530 milligrams (mg) of valerian root daily for one month can lead to improvements in sleep quality and shorten the time it takes a person to fall asleep. Short-term use of valerian root appears to be safe for adults, but the safety remains uncertain for long-term use.

Magnesium

Magnesium is a mineral found in the body and in many foods, including dried beans and legumes, dark green leafy vegetables, and nuts, such as almonds and cashews. Magnesium can have a relaxing effect on the muscles of the body and appears to have a calming effect on the brain by increasing levels of a neurotransmitter called gamma-amino-butyric acid (GABA). One small study showed a positive effect on sleep when 175 milligrams (mg) of magnesium was combined with both melatonin and vitamin B complex. A common recommended dose for magnesium is up to 225 mg.

Tryptophan

Tryptophan is an essential *amnio acid* (a molecule that joins with other amino acids to form proteins) that performs many functions in the body. It aids in the production of a neurotransmitter called serotonin, which is a brain chemical that affects mood and sleep. At night, serotonin helps produce melatonin. (See how all these things in your body are connected?)

Tryptophan naturally occurs in many foods, including shellfish, soy products, seeds, nuts, and turkey. (Remember that feeling of exhaustion after eating that Thanksgiving dinner?)

No studies show that the amount of tryptophan present in foods has a consistent positive or negative effect on sleep or moods, but some small studies that have inconsistent results show that taking it as a supplement may help insomnia. (By the way, a lot of other factors at the Thanksgiving dinner table that can make you sleepy, such as all those carbs — don't be so quick to blame the turkey!)

Improving sleep by using hormones

Because one of the reasons for poor sleep in perimenopause probably involves a rapid change in hormone levels, you may think that the solution involves taking hormones. However, no studies have shown that hormones can work as a sleep aid, and insomnia alone usually doesn't suggest to your doctor that you should start a hormone program. However, you may find that taking hormones for other symptoms, such as hot flashes and night sweats, may also result in a better night's sleep.

Progesterone

Progesterone, a naturally occurring hormone produced in the ovaries of reproductive-age women, is present in many biological activities in the body. It affects mood, breathing, appetite, memory, and sexual activity. It also can exert a sleep induction or hypnotic effect on the body.

While you age, hormone levels, including progesterone, fluctuate and then begin to decline. If your sleep issues are caused in part by low or fluctuating progesterone levels, then replacing the missing progesterone may be very effective in restoring the calm relaxation needed for better sleep.

Progestin, although its name sounds similar to progesterone, isn't a natural hormone; it's a synthetic chemical that can mimic the effects of progesterone in the body. Several different types of progestin are manufactured in the lab, and although progestin may work similarly in the body to progesterone, each type of synthetic progestin has its own effects on the body.

You need to take supplemental progesterone/progestin orally to see an effect on your sleep patterns. Using progesterone in a cream or a vaginal suppository probably doesn't offer any benefits to sleep.

Micronized progesterone has proven very safe and has few side effects. You can get it with a prescription, and it comes in strengths of 100 milligrams (mg) or 200 mg. You usually take a single dose at bedtime, and you may have to wait several weeks to have a sleep-inducing effect.

Some common side effects include

>> Breast tenderness

>> Headaches

>> Dizziness

>> Drowsiness

Estrogen

Estrogen fluctuates during perimenopause and ultimately declines while your ovaries age. If you have trouble sleeping through the night because of your body's inability to regulate your nighttime body temperature (resulting in night sweats), adding estrogen into your perimenopausal sleep plan may help.

If your healthcare provider and you rule out other causes of nighttime sweating (such as infection, thyroid abnormalities, or too much alcohol before bed), if you haven't already, consult a gynecologist who specializes in perimenopausal hormone management to help you relieve the nighttime sweats. The two of you can come up with a personalized plan that includes appropriate and safe estrogen doses, which can eliminate those nighttime flashes and help you get a good night of sleep.

Finding a nap app to send you to dreamland

You can find many sleep apps on the market that are designed to help you fall asleep and stay asleep:

>> **White noise:** Block out noises that can keep you awake by introducing constant, soothing sound.

>> **Relaxation:** Help you relax so that you can get to sleep.

>> **Sleep trackers:** Aim to chart and document your sleep patterns, such as how long it takes you to fall asleep and how long you remain in the various stages of sleep.

You can use some of these apps for free, but some are quite expensive and work on a subscription model. Sleep apps are quite popular and easy to use (for the most part) — people have downloaded them millions of times in the past ten years.

If you do try a sleep app, keep your phone face down so that the light from the screen doesn't disturb your sleep. (See the advice in the section "Improving sleep hygiene," earlier in this chapter — no looking at cellphones before bed.)

Apps that block noise

Blocking out annoying noises and replacing them with soothing music or white noise, such as the sound of ocean waves, tapping, or a steadily moving train, can help you sleep better. Most white noise apps give you a variety of sounds to try out to see whether a particular noise improves your ability to fall asleep.

Apps designed for mental relaxation

Most relaxation apps utilize soothing voices that offer some form of meditation or guided imagery. Sometimes, a calming voice describes peaceful scenes, occasionally accompanied by music.

You can also find sleep hypnosis apps, and although clinical studies are scanty, some people feel that these apps can improve quality and length of sleep.

Apps that track your sleep

Several apps can track your sleep habits via a wearable device. These apps collect data about how long it takes you to fall asleep, how long you spend in the deeper stages of sleep, and how much you move around in your sleep. Experts say that sleep tracker apps can help make you more aware of your sleep patterns and potentially help correct some problematic sleep habits. However, these sleep trackers aren't always accurate, and you can't use them to diagnose a sleep disorder.

ORTHOSOMNIA AND THE CASE AGAINST SLEEP TRACKERS

The more we understand about the value of healthy sleep patterns and the benefits of sleep to our health and wellbeing, the more many people go to great efforts in pursuit of the perfect night's sleep — characterized by duration, schedule consistency, and overall quality. In 2017, researchers at Rush University Medical School and Northwestern University's Feinberg School of Medicine actually coined the phrased "orthosomnia" to describe people who become overly preoccupied with regularly getting the perfect sleep.

Tracking technology is used by millions to monitor (and optimize) sleep patterns. Apps on phones and watches are able to monitor biometric data, movement, and even record noise as you sleep. You can set your smart phone or watch to remind you to wind down and go to bed.

But the use of such tools has been shown to backfire, actually causing a decline in sleep quality. For one, keeping devices like phones and smart watches out of the bedroom has been shown to improve sleep. But also, becoming consumed with perfect sleep, for many, causes stress and anxiety that leads to sleep disturbances.

Obsessive monitoring (constantly checking sleep data, such as sleep duration, sleep stages, and other metrics) and insisting on rigid sleep schedules (which can be limited, for example at the expense of social engagements) can cause individuals to experience:

Anxiety and stress: They may experience heightened anxiety and stress related to achieving a certain quantity or quality of sleep.

Difficulty falling (and staying) asleep: The pressure to achieve perfect sleep can lead to difficulty falling asleep due to heightened stress levels.

Worsened sleep quality: The obsession with achieving perfect sleep can lead to poorer sleep quality, as the stress and anxiety associated with these efforts can disrupt natural sleep patterns.

Several patients have reported to me that they actually got worse sleep after getting a sleep tracker. When talking about why they felt the tracker had a detrimental effect on their sleep, they all mentioned that looking at their sleep statistics made them so anxious that they stayed up at night worrying about what their reports would reveal about their sleep habits the next morning. The app was adding to their stress, not reducing it. If you find yourself in this camp, definitely stop using the app. If it's not helping, it's not useful.

Using prescription sleep medications

If you regularly have insomnia, and no options from the recommendations I suggest in the preceding sections have helped, you may want to consider a prescription sleep aid. Certain sleeping pills may help when temporary conditions, such as stress, travel, or other disruptions, are keeping you awake. Some sleep aids can help you fall asleep; some can help you stay asleep. All prescription sleep medications have risks, and many of them can lead to dependence.

Drugs that your doctor might prescribe for sleep include the medications listed in Table 11-1.

TABLE 11-1

Medications to Treat Insomnia

Medication	Brand Name	Drug Type	Risk of Dependence
Doxepin	Silenor	Tricyclic antidepressant	Low
Amitriptyline	Elavil	Tricyclic antidepressant	Low
Mirtazapine	Remeron	Tetracyclic antidepressant	Low
Trazodone	Desyrel	SARI antidepressant	Low
Ramelteon	Rozerem	CNS depressant	Low
Zolpidem	Ambien	Sedative/hypnotic	High
Zaleplon	Sonata	Sedative/hypnotic	High
Eszopiclone	Lunesta	Sedative/hypnotic	High
Temazepam	Restoril	Benzodiazepine	High

All of the medications in Table 11-1 have the potential side effects of dizziness and nausea.

The antidepressant medications in Table 11-1 aren't addictive and may prevent age-related cognitive decline. However, they have potential side effects:

>> Fatigue

>> Dry mouth

>> Weakness

>> Irritability

All of the medications that have a high risk of dependence in Table 11-1 can have additional side effects, including

>> Headaches

>> Changes in thinking and behavior

>> Memory and performance problems

WARNING

You may have heard stories of people who got out of bed, ate large meals, drove their cars, and afterward had no recollection of these activities while they were under the influence of certain sleep-aid medications. Relying on these medications for long periods of time increases the likelihood of negative side effects. Taking sleep-aid medications can increase your risk for falls and accidents, as well as increasing the risk for dementia in older populations. If you have to take a sleep-aid medication, do so for only a short period of time, usually between two weeks and two months.

REMEMBER

If your medical provider can identify an underlying cause for the sleep disruptions, treating that medical condition or sleep-related disorder can provide the most effective therapy.

Trying over-the-counter sleep aids

Some over-the-counter (OTC) sleep aids may be worth a try. Common over-the-counter sleep aids include these sedating antihistamines (which can cause daytime drowsiness, dry mouth, and constipation):

>> Diphenhydramine

>> Doxylamine

Combination products that include acetaminophen or ibuprofen, along with diphenhydramine, provide the combined benefit of pain relief and better sleep; some products also combine acetaminophen with doxylamine and dextromethorphan (a cough suppressant).

If you want to try an OTC sleep aid, here's some information to arm you:

>> Most sleep aids available without a prescription contain an antihistamine or a supplement, such as melatonin (which you can read about in the section "Melatonin," earlier in this chapter).

>> Some may have a combination of supplements or various medications: Read the labels to find out what exactly you're taking.

>> Tolerance to the sedative effects of OTC antihistamines can develop quickly; if you take them for a long period of time, they're less likely to work.

>> Some of these medications can leave you feeling like you have a hangover the next morning: groggy and unwell, with a headache.

>> The medications in a sleep aid may interact with or increase the potency of other medications that you take. Check for drug interactions with your doctor.

TIP

Always read the labels. You can accidentally take an unsafe amount of any of these medications, even though they're sold over the counter.

Seeking the help of a sleep specialist

Imagine seeing a medical professional whose only job is to help you have better sleep! A *sleep specialist* is an expert in medicine who has been specially trained in sleep disorders.

Sleep disorders have their own diagnostic criteria, and they can have a profound effect on the quality of your life. The first step to dealing with any sleep disorder is getting an appropriate diagnosis. A sleep specialist is the professional most likely to diagnose, explain, and treat your sleep disorder effectively.

In perimenopause, because of several factors (fluctuating hormones, high stress levels, changing family situations, mood disorders, disruptions in bleeding patterns, and physical changes), good quality sleep takes a nosedive. Poor sleep can make you feel unfocused and lead to other, more severe medical and health problems. If you have symptoms of a major sleep disorder, you may want to seek professional help.

If you have any of the following symptoms, consider seeing a sleep specialist:

>> **Chronic insomnia:** Not remedied by any lifestyle changes, supplements, or medications that I discuss throughout this chapter, and not explained by other treatable medical conditions.

>> **Sleep apnea:** Where sleep is disrupted by breathing issues during the night.

>> **Severe drowsiness:** Falling asleep during the day; inability to concentrate or work because of extreme tiredness.

>> **Restless legs:** An irresistible urge to move your legs while at rest; this symptom can happen in the daytime or nighttime. Flip to the section "Restless leg syndrome," earlier in this chapter, for more details.

4

Maintaining a Healthy Body

IN THIS CHAPTER

» Looking at how the urinary tract works

» Understanding the bladder at midlife

» Examining the different types of incontinence

» Seeking to regain control of your bladder

Chapter **12**

Managing a Bladder That Won't Behave

The very first time it happens, you may look around to see whether anyone noticed. Maybe you're standing in the backyard at your sister's barbeque, sneeze a giant sneeze, and feel a small (or a large) gush. "Was that . . . pee?" you say to yourself (horrified). And, depending on what you're wearing and how big of a gush, you may finish your conversation, or you may make a run for the house, backing your way into the bathroom to investigate.

That scenario presents an episode of bladder leakage, also called *incontinence*, and it's another one of those inconvenient, unwelcome, and sometimes surprising bodily changes that you may experience while you transition through perimenopause.

These years of perimenopause may remind you of your teen years, where periods and emotions were also out of control. Where the bladder is concerned, it may remind you of an even earlier time — when you were four and had a hard time "holding it" because the signal to pee may have come too late for you to recognize it. In perimenopause, the leak may return, but it need not destroy your quality of (mid)life.

In this chapter, I talk about bladder control — and lack of control. You can find out a bit about the anatomy and physiology of the urinary tract. This chapter also discusses which solutions can help which bladder problems so that you can take control of your bladder function.

Understanding the Normal Function of the Urinary Tract

So, what's causing this bladder leakage, and when and how can you stop it? If you want answers to the latter, and no doubt most important, question, check out the section "Seeking Treatment (and Relief!)" later in this chapter. In this section, you can take a look at how your bladder — shown in Figure 12-1 — and the entire urinary system is designed to function.

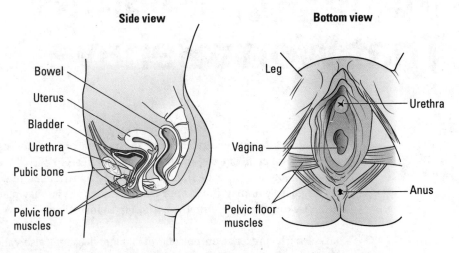

Side view

Bowel

Uterus

Bladder

Urethra

Pubic bone

Pelvic floor muscles

Bottom view

Leg

Urethra

Vagina

Anus

Pelvic floor muscles

FIGURE 12-1:
The bladder, urethra and pelvic organs.

>> **Kidneys:** Bean-shaped organs located in your lower back area that remove waste and extra fluid from your body, as well as maintaining the balance of *electrolytes* — minerals such as sodium, calcium, phosphorus, and potassium — in your blood.

Kidneys themselves aren't affected or changed much when the body goes through perimenopause for perimenopause-specific reasons. But they are organs, and while all organs get older, they may work less efficiently.

>> **Ureters:** Each kidney — most people have two, although your body can usually operate with only one — drains via a tube called the *ureter* into the urinary bladder, which acts as a temporary storage reservoir for urine.

>> **Bladder:** Located just behind your pubic bone and right in front of the uterus. It's kind of like an elastic balloon and expands when it fills up. In a typical adult, this balloon can hold between 200 and 400 milliliters (mL) of urine before you feel an urge to urinate. However, a bladder can sometimes hold much more or much less, depending on its health and elasticity. (For comparison, 500mL is the amount in half of a 1-liter soda bottle.)

Nerves in the bladder wall detect the bladder's expansion and send a signal to the brain, letting it know that the bladder is full. When you voluntarily empty your bladder, the muscle in the bladder wall contracts and tightens to squeeze the urine out of your bladder. Although this contraction of bladder wall muscle is happening, the muscle at the base of the bladder needs to relax so that the bladder can empty.

>> **Urethra:** A small tube that connects the bladder to the outside, through which urine flows.

If any part of this pathway isn't working properly, then your bladder may not function properly, resulting in various types of leaking and incontinence. Here are some potential culprits behind bladder malfunction:

>> **Bladder:** May not expand properly or enough

>> **Nerves in the bladder walls:** May not be working effectively enough to sense fullness

>> **Signal to the brain:** May not effectively alert you to a sense of fullness

>> **Bladder muscles:** May not be able to contract and squeeze adequately to empty the bladder at the appropriate time (such as when you're sitting on the toilet)

>> **Muscle at the base of the bladder:** May not relax, relaxes too much, or relaxes at the wrong time to allow urine to flow

You may be able to control some of these issues on your own, and you can probably fix others by using certain medical treatments.

Midlife Bladder: Why Is This Happening Now?

Hormonal changes that accompany perimenopause in midlife, as well as child-bearing in earlier years, affect components of the urinary tract:

>> **Hormone fluctuation:** Estrogen levels can vary widely at this time, and the *urethra* (the tube through which urine flows out of your body) is very sensitive to those changes. When estrogen levels drop, the muscles around the urethra are less efficient, and emptying can become problematic. Those tissues around the urethra become thinner and less elastic, so small tears can occur, which allow bacteria to enter the urethra, causing inflammation, infection, pain, and leakage.

>> **Weight gain:** Also, midlife is a time when many women gain some weight, often around the midsection. Carrying extra weight in the midsection of your body can increase your chances of experiencing urinary incontinence by putting more pressure on the bladder. A study done in 2011 concluded that women who lost 5 to 10 percent of their body weight had significant reductions in urinary incontinence.

>> **Previous childbirth:** By the time they hit perimenopause, many women have gone through childbirth, which can cause damage to the pelvic floor, worsening bladder function. Depending on the number of deliveries, the size of the babies, and the length of time pushing during delivery, the muscles and ligaments surrounding the bladder and urethra may have weakened, allowing more leakage to occur. (Unfortunately, having Cesarean section deliveries doesn't guarantee no later-on leaks.)

Evaluating Incontinence

Any degree of urine leakage is termed *incontinence*, but not all incontinence is the same:

>> **An underlying issue:** Your incontinence may be temporary, caused by vaginal dryness, infection, or tissue damage. When you resolve the underlying problem, the incontinence may go away.

>> **Age-related:** You may notice your incontinence worsening over time; a little leakage can become a lot of leakage while you get older. This type of incontinence likely doesn't go away on its own. You can speak with your healthcare provider about possible treatments.

>> **Anatomical problems:** Some urinary incontinence occurs because of problems of anatomy, and some may be caused by nerve damage or dysfunction.

You and your doctor need to identify the type (or types) of incontinence that you're experiencing to find a solution.

Stress incontinence

Stress incontinence occurs when you laugh, cough, sneeze, run, jump, or pick up something heavy and your body releases anything from a trickle to a large gush of urine right then. Yes, this type of incontinence *is* stressful, but the name of this type of incontinence refers to the abdominal pressure that's created when coughing, laughing, jumping, or lifting. That pressure is stronger than the pressure at the closed urethra, so the urethra is forced to open, causing leakage. These factors can lead to weakened pelvic floor muscles:

>> Childbirth

>> Injuries to the area around the bladder or the urethra

>> Some medications

>> Surgery to the area

This type of incontinence has to do with your anatomy; the muscles in the area surrounding the bladder and the urethra (the *pelvic floor*) aren't strong enough to keep that urethra closed when they encounter a sudden rise in pressure. In the section "Strengthening those pelvic muscles," later in the chapter, I discuss some options that you have.

Urge incontinence

Urge incontinence occurs when the nerve signals between the brain and the bladder aren't working properly. You may feel the sudden urge to urinate and just can't make it to the bathroom in time. You may feel uncomfortable muscle spasms in the bladder (but not always), and you may get up multiple times in the middle of the night to urinate. This form of incontinence is also called *overactive bladder*.

Mixed incontinence

When you have elements of both stress and urge incontinence (see the preceding sections), doctors call that *mixed incontinence*. So you experience an urge to urinate, resulting in random leakage, and then you have additional leakage when you cough, sneeze, or do anything that increases your intra-abdominal pressure. See your healthcare provider so that they can evaluate your incontinence problems and treat the issue or issues to stop (or lessen) the leaks.

URINARY TRACT INFECTIONS AND INCONTINENCE

Urinary tract infections (UTI) happen when bacteria that lives outside or near the bladder or urethra somehow makes their way into the urinary tract. These bacteria can affect the urethra, bladder, and even the kidneys if they travel up through the urinary system. The most common place for a UTI is in the bladder (also called *cystitis*). Wiping after you urinate may actually move bacteria from the skin and the vaginal area right into the urethra. The urethra in women is fairly short (about 4 cm in length, or 1.5 in.), which gives this wiped bacteria a point of access. Also, the urethra is very close to the vaginal opening, and during perimenopause, the vagina may become drier and its tissues thinner. Bacteria can easily migrate from the vagina into the urethra during sexual activity.

UTIs usually have very specific and recognizable symptoms: burning, frequent urination, pain, muscle spasms when attempting to urinate, or blood in the urine. Some women may also suddenly have random leakage.

You healthcare provider can treat urinary tract infections by prescribing antibiotics. When the lab identifies a specific bacteria on a urine test (also called a *urine culture*), your doctor can prescribe an antibiotic that treats that particular type of bacteria.

You can also take medications to help ease the pain of a urinary tract infection, called analgesics. Some prescription analgesics sometimes change the color of your urine to orange or blue, depending on which one you use. Analgesics don't treat a urinary tract infection because they don't include antibiotics.

Although you can find many home remedies suggested for urinary tract infections, most have no clear evidence that they treat infections, including taking vitamin C, cranberry juice, eating cranberries, taking probiotics, and using feminine wipes. Don't use these methods and delay seeking medical treatments that can help resolve the infection and ease your pain.

Overflow incontinence

When you have *overflow incontinence*, you experience frequent or constant dribbling of urine because your bladder doesn't empty completely. You may have the urge to urinate but only release a small amount when you sit down to go. This kind of incontinence can be caused by nerve or muscle damage, or certain neurological conditions. Often, addressing the underlying medical, physical, or neurological condition can help lessen or stop this type of leakage.

INTERSTITIAL CYSTITIS: AN OFTEN-UNDIAGNOSED PROBLEM

Interstitial cystitis (IC) is a very specific and underdiagnosed bladder condition. Symptoms are very similar to a urinary tract infection (burning, pain, spasms of the urethra, difficulty emptying), but test after test of the urine come back as negative for infection. The average age of a woman who has interstitial cystitis is 42. Doctors don't know whether hormonal changes may play a role in IC, and for a diagnosis of IC, a physician needs to take a look inside the bladder with a camera, called a *cystoscope.* By using a cystoscope, the doctor can see whether the interior of your bladder has any microscopic tears, inflammation, or other findings to explain the symptoms.

Treatments for IC range from least invasive (modifying your diet) to the most invasive (bladder surgery). Some women find that eliminating certain foods and drinks from the diet, such as alcohol, caffeine, sharp cheeses, acidic foods, and artificial sweeteners helps to relieve bladder irritation. You also can find several medications in use for the treatment of interstitial cystitis. Only one is made specifically for IC — pentosan polysulfate (brand name Elmiron). This medication has actually been found to repair some of the damage to the bladder wall that occurs when you have this condition. Other medications are used *off label* (meaning to treat a condition other than the condition the drug has been approved for) to manage the pain of IC: Antidepressants, antihistamines, and analgesics have all shown some benefit for long-term management, usually along with dietary changes. Surgery for IC is rare and usually involves some type of repair to the bladder walls by a specialist in bladder surgery, called a *urologist.*

Seeking Treatment (and Relief!)

If all of the potential problems outlined in the section "Evaluating Incontinence," earlier in this chapter, sound terribly grim, don't despair. You can often treat or mitigate these bladder issues through various interventions. The approach that you take to alleviate your bladder issues depends on the causes, the length of time it's been a problem, and your overall general health.

If you're having incontinence issues, see a doctor who specializes in urinary tract conditions (a urologist or a gynecologist); but if that's not an option, many primary care providers can also evaluate you and start a workup for complaints of leakage or urgency. Incontinence may be a sign of a serious medical condition such as diabetes, multiple sclerosis, or a stroke, so your doctor needs to eliminate these potential causes before you both can decide on some treatment options.

Strengthening those pelvic muscles

For stress incontinence caused by pelvic floor muscle weakness, you can do pelvic floor exercises, known as *Kegel muscles,* at home or as taught by a pelvic floor physical therapist. Pelvic floor physical therapy is a specialized form of physical therapy (PT) that focuses on the muscles of the pelvic floor. This kind of PT usually includes retraining and strengthening the muscles that control bowel and bladder function. Your pelvic floor PT may also evaluate and treat your back, hips, abdomen, and pelvis, working on the areas needed to improve function and reduce leakage.

You can also purchase devices to help strengthen your pelvic floor; some devices even have apps that can teach you how to best utilize the devices. These devices range in price from a few hundred dollars to a few thousand dollars and have varying degrees of success. Little research exists on these gadgets.

>> **Biofeedback:** Most of these devices work by having you place a biofeedback device in the vagina, which helps to direct your Kegel.

>> **Electrical stimulation:** Some devices use electrical stimulation to cause vaginal and pelvic floor muscles to contract. (They do your Kegel exercises for you.) These devices can help you add strength to very lax muscles.

REMEMBER

Prior to using any home-based electrical devices, get an evaluation by a physician or a pelvic floor therapist to make sure that the device will treat the problem that you have. You may have symptoms that sound like someone else's, but yours may be a very different problem.

>> **Weights:** You insert Kegel exercise weights (which come in various shapes, sizes, and weights) into the vagina and do guided exercises to help strengthen and train the pelvic floor muscles.

Using these weights incorrectly or for too long can cause muscle spasms and worsen incontinence or pain.

WARNING

ENHANCING STRENGTH WITH KEGEL EXERCISES: A SIMPLE THREE-STEP ROUTINE

Kegel exercises are performed by lifting, holding, and then relaxing your pelvic floor muscles.

Start by locating your pelvic floor muscles. To find your pelvic floor muscles, try stopping the flow of urine when you are sitting on the toilet. Only do this in order to locate these muscles and to see how it feels. You can also imagine that you are trying to prevent yourself from allowing gas to pass. Or, you can try inserting a finger (or a device made specifically for safely doing Kegel exercises) into the vagina, and squeezing your vaginal muscles around it. It should feel like there is a circle, closing around the finger or device, and "lifting" it into the pelvis. These are the same muscles that you will use during Kegel exercises.

You perform these exercises by lifting and holding for a period of time (usually just a few seconds to start) and then relaxing the pelvic floor muscles. Start by doing a few at a time, then gradually increase the strength and the length of time as well as the number of repetitions that you are doing in each session. You should do at least two to three sets of these exercises per day.

1. Lying down on your back, first locate your pelvic floor muscles.

2. Start by tightening your pelvic floor muscles for 3 seconds, then relax for 3 seconds. This is one Kegel. You may be slightly lifting your bottom off the ground, but do not use the butt or leg muscles; this is for the vaginal/pelvic muscles to tighten and lift toward the inside of your body.

3. Repeat this ten times. This is one set.

(continued)

(continued)

4. Do one set every morning and one at night.

5. Increase the number of repetitions, and the length of time you hold each contraction until you are doing three sets of ten, holding each for 5-7 seconds.

Doing Kegels correctly should not hurt your stomach, abdominal muscles, lower back, or head. If you are holding your breath or clenching the wrong muscles, you may start to have some of these side effects.

You can tell that you are making improvements if there are fewer incidents of leakage when you cough, sneeze, run, or lift something heavy.

You can improve the strength of your Kegel after several weeks by moving from the lying down position to sitting up and then standing. If you have trouble getting started with these exercises on your own, it may be a good idea to ask your doctor to refer you to a pelvic floor physical therapist to teach you the proper way to use these muscles, before continuing to do them at home.

When doing a regular Kegel exercise program at home, you should begin to see changes in 6 to 8 weeks.

TIP

If you need to stop incontinence by using a temporary measure, consider these devices:

>> **Incontinence tampons:** Intravaginal mechanical devices designed for women who have stress incontinence in very specific situations. These devices look similar to tampons for menstrual flow, but after you insert them into your vagina, they open up into a shape that places pressure on the urethra. This helps to stop leakage during physical stress such as running or hiking. It comes in three sizes, and you shouldn't wear one for more than 12 hours at a time.

>> **Vaginal pessary:** A vaginal device made of plastic that you can place in the vagina and leave in place for longer than the 12 hours approved for incontinence tampons. It gently puts pressure on the urethra, which improves the support of the urethra and reduces urinary leakage. (See sidebar for more information on this.)

HOW A VAGINAL PESSARY IS FITTED

A pessary is a device that is designed to fit inside the vaginal canal, for women who have a prolapse (descent) of the uterus, bladder wall, vaginal walls, or rectum. A pessary is fitted in a doctor's office and must fit well to provide relief and to be safe. A well-fitting pessary can help decrease the symptoms of prolapse, prevent a prolapse from worsening, help avoid or delay surgery for prolapse, and provide temporary relief from urinary leakage. A well-fitting pessary sits comfortably inside the vagina when you are sitting, lying down, or standing upright. It should stay in place when you empty your bladder, and not cause an inability to empty. It should not keep you from emptying your bowels and should not fall out when you are urinating or having a bowel movement. If it moves around within the vaginal canal, causing irritation, you may need to be refitted, as the size may be too big or too small or the shape may be wrong. There should be no bleeding, no discharge, no pain, or signs of infection while the pessary is in place, and it should be removed, cleaned, and reinserted based on the schedule that is acceptable to you and your healthcare provider.

Surgery and procedures for stress incontinence

Several options exist for surgical solutions to stress leakage (but definitely have extensive conversations with your doctor to confirm that surgery is the right decision for you):

>> **Sling placement:** The most common procedure is placement of a sling. A surgeon (usually a urologist, a gynecologist, or a specialized combination of these two, called a urogynecologist) uses the patient's own tissue, synthetic material (mesh), or animal or donor tissue to create a sling or a hammock that supports the urethra. The midurethral sling is the most common type of sling placed.

>> **Colposuspension:** Utilizes an abdominal incision to lift the neck of the bladder and stitch it into this lifted and elevated position. The surgeon conducts this surgery either through an abdominal incision or a *laparoscopy* (where they insert a small camera into the abdomen through a small incision, and they perform the surgery through other small incisions).

>> **Injections:** A doctor injects synthetic material into the tissues that surround the urethra to bulk them up and help support the weakened muscles. This minor procedure can usually be done in an office setting and by using local anesthesia. Sometimes, your doctor needs to do multiple injections to get the desired result.

The type of surgery that you have depends on many factors, including age, future childbearing plans, lifestyle, medical history, general health, and the cause of the problem.

Medications for overactive bladders

No matter how many pelvic floor exercises you do or how many devices you try (see the section "Strengthening those pelvic muscles," earlier in this chapter), if you have overactive bladder (which I discuss in the section "Urge incontinence," earlier in this chapter), they can't help. Because this type of incontinence is caused by nerves signaling improperly or by irritated muscles, the treatments must address these problems. Have you ever seen a TV commercial where a woman is being "led around" by her (cartoon) bladder, which happens to always be walking alongside her, in the mall, at dinner, and in the park? This is a clever way to ask whether your bladder is always controlling you — making you seek out the closest bathroom, coordinate your timing so that you won't leak before you get there. Of course, that commercial was an advertisement for a medication that you can take to relieve your overactive bladder symptoms. You can find many different medications available to treat overactive bladder, all with various success rates, side effects, and costs.

Some of these medications, which work by relaxing the muscles in the wall of the bladder, include

>> Fesoterodine (brand name Toviaz)

>> Mirabegron (brand name Myrbetriq)

>> Oxybutynin (brand name Oxytrol)

>> Solifenacin (brand name Vesicare)

>> Tolterodine (brand name Detrol)

Before you can start taking one of these medications, your healthcare provider needs to evaluate you to determine which medication best fits your diagnosis. Your doctor will probably do a physical exam, a urinalysis, and sometimes a series of tests called *urodynamics*. Urodynamic studies

>> Assess the function of your bladder muscles.

>> Check how completely you can empty your bladder.

>> Test your bladder pressure to identify any involuntary muscle contractions or problems with urine storage.

Urodynamic testing may feel a little strange because, essentially, you have to fill your bladder and then urinate while someone watches, measures, and documents it.

WARNING

Medications that help relieve urge incontinence usually have side effects such as dry eyes, dry mouth, and constipation. The same way that they dry the bladder, they may also dry the rest of you, so treat these side effects if they occur by using eye drops and stool softeners.

Nerve stimulation

To relieve the symptoms of overactive bladder, your doctor might recommend nerve stimulation. This treatment regulates nerve impulses to the bladder, in one of several ways:

» **Wire-implant surgical procedure:** A surgeon places a thin wire close to the sacral nerves in the lower back. These nerves carry signals to your bladder. After a temporary trial, and if all goes well, the surgeon can place this wire permanently. You use a hand-held device to deliver electrical impulses to your bladder. Sounds kind of painful, but you don't actually feel a thing. The success rate of these implants is pretty high, with about 50 to 80-percent improvement in bladder leakage symptoms.

» **Percutaneous tibial nerve stimulation (PTNS):** A procedure done in an office setting where a doctor places a thin needle through the skin near your ankle attached to an electronic device that sends electrical stimulation from the nerve in your leg (the *tibial nerve*) to your spine, where it connects with nerves that control the bladder. You receive these treatments once a week for 12 weeks, and then you have them monthly for maintenance therapy to keep symptoms under control.

» **Bladder injections:** These injections can help severe urge incontinence (which I talk about in the section "Urge incontinence," earlier in this chapter). Just like people use Botox to get rid of wrinkles, a doctor can inject Botox directly into the bladder tissues to relax them. This injection can relieve urge incontinence, but the effects are usually temporary. Although it can last up to six months, you still need to get repeat injections after the effects wear off.

WARNING

These injections can cause a serious side effect called *urinary retention,* which is a complete inability to urinate. You may need to use a *urinary catheter* (a tube inserted in the urethra to drain the bladder) in the worst cases.

For mixed incontinence, which may have elements of both stress and urge incontinence (see the section "Mixed incontinence," earlier in this chapter), you may need a combination of treatments for each type.

Behavioral techniques for relieving your bladder symptoms

After your doctor takes a full history and evaluates you to determine reasons for your incontinence, they may have various suggestions and recommendations that you can follow to stop your leaks. Here's a list of behavioral techniques that may also help you while you're being evaluated or while you're awaiting your appointments for further workup:

>> **Bladder training:** This method of training involves trying to delay urination when you first get the urge to go. You can start by holding off for five or ten minutes every time you feel the need to urinate. Lengthen the delay weekly until intervals between urinating are 2.5 to 3 hours.

>> **Double voiding:** Helps to empty the bladder more completely to avoid it ever getting overly full and causing overflow incontinence. With this technique, after you urinate, even if you feel like you've completely emptied your bladder, wait another few minutes and try again. (Don't push the urine out — urinate because the muscles relax.)

>> **Scheduled toilet trips:** Urinate on a schedule; set a timer and urinate every 2.5 to 4 hours, instead of waiting for the urge to go.

>> **Managing your fluids and your diet:** Certain foods and drinks irritate the bladder. Cutting down on alcohol, caffeine, and acidic foods may help to decrease leakage and bladder discomfort. Reducing the total amount of liquid you consume in a day, losing weight, and increasing physical activity for overall health can all improve bladder function and reduce leakage.

>> **Treating vaginal dryness:** During perimenopause, the lack of continuous estrogen affects all the areas of your body that have estrogen receptors. The vagina is in close proximity to the urethra and the bladder, so when the vagina is dry, it affects the surrounding tissues, as well. Moisturizers, as well as vaginally applied estrogen and other hormones, can improve the elasticity and health of the genital area and improve bladder function, as well.

Chapter **13**

Maintaining a Healthy Diet Before Menopause

D on't believe the idea that the years of midlife automatically come with a laundry list of health problems and medical conditions. You can take control of your health at any time. And with menopause looming, the time to establish (and continue) good and healthy lifestyle habits is now! The more you can incorporate healthy eating and healthy movement into your everyday life, the more easily you can maintain those habits into your later years.

In this chapter, you can find out how to minimize health risks prior to menopause by finding nutritional and lifestyle plans that you can easily incorporate into your daily life. I offer some information to help you formulate a healthy eating plan that you can stick to forever. Also, you can pick from a list of exercises in Chapter 14 that can help you to live your best and healthiest life.

Staying Healthy for Life

Researchers have determined that the habits you must have to live a long and healthy life include these five things:

» Maintain a healthy body weight (I talk about weight in the section "Managing Weight," later in this chapter).

» Eat a high-quality diet (see the following section, as well as the sections "Getting the Right Mix of Nutrients" and "Eating for strong bones," later in this chapter, for tips on a healthy perimenopause eating plan).

» Exercise at least at a moderate pace most days of the week (flip to Chapter 14 for more on exercise).

» Don't smoke.

» Limit your alcohol intake; no more than three alcoholic beverages per week.

Eating for the Change

Starting in your midlife years, you experience many subtle (and some not-so-subtle) physical reminders that your body is changing. An extra glass of wine, or having a daily bowl of ice cream, may start to affect your body differently than it did when you were in your 20s or 30s.

Although you may find this new reality disappointing, you can also try to look at it as a wakeup call, a welcome signal that you may need to change some of your habits and take this opportunity for a bit of course correction. Fluctuating hormone levels, especially estrogen, may increase your risk of medical conditions such as heart disease and osteoporosis, but a healthy diet can help lower these risks and give you better energy, sleep, and emotional stability.

You do have to pay attention to what you eat and how you eat during perimenopause. Even if, in your youth, you were that lucky person who could eat whatever you wanted and drink alcohol regularly without suffering the weight-related consequences, that likely starts to change in perimenopause. Weight that shifts to your middle, pounds that accumulate with no major change in your diet, and clothes that no longer fit may become the norm.

Develop healthy habits that become as much of a daily routine as brushing your teeth and that don't feel like tremendous sacrifices so that those healthy eating habits and healthy choices can guide you for the rest of your life.

Keep your goals in mind

Establish a perimenopausal transition diet to

>> Provide yourself maximal protection from diseases and medical problems.

>> Boost your energy.

>> Help with good restorative sleep.

>> Maintain a healthy weight.

A balanced diet of food and drink can keep your body well-nourished and help to avoid many medical conditions that relate to dietary intake, such as diabetes and heart disease. A mix of healthy foods can help provide protection to your heart and blood vessels, lower your risk of certain cancers, and improve your body's immune function (which boosts your body's ability to fight off certain illnesses and infections).

Eating healthy includes some basic rules and suggestions. You don't have to count every calorie or use some complicated formula to make sure that you get enough of the nutrients your body needs. But in general, you need to:

>> Take in the right proportions of carbohydrates, fats, and proteins (see the section "Getting the Right Mix of Nutrients," later in this chapter).

>> Have a daily calorie intake that isn't more than your expenditure.

>> Focus on nutrient-dense, healthy foods.

>> Limit consumption of alcohol and eliminate highly processed and packaged foods.

>> Generally practice mindful, distraction-free eating; try to eat mostly at the table, not in the car, on the run, or in front of the refrigerator.

>> Recognize disordered eating, such as emotional eating, extreme dieting, and binge eating If you have this kind of eating problem, seek professional help.

REMEMBER

Fad diets and trendy diets come and go. Please ignore them. Don't think of your eating plan as a diet where you need to eliminate certain food groups or eat from only certain food groups to stay healthy. You need food not just for survival, but also for enjoyment. A well-balanced, healthy diet can keep you full, healthy, and satisfied. Eating with a purpose (your health and satisfaction) can fuel your body and mind and keep all your moving parts functioning efficiently.

Identifying social and emotional eating

People eat for a lot of reasons other than to satisfy hunger. As a matter of fact, many people don't really know how to identify hunger.

Any number of emotions and situations can trigger you to eat. You may eat

>> For comfort

>> For social reasons

>> Out of boredom, anger, anxiety, or sadness

>> In celebration

Sometimes, you eat just because you have the food (and the company) in front of you; at a party or an event, the food is plentiful and looks so good.

If you can separate all the other reasons for eating and start to listen to your hunger cues, you can make your eating more purposeful.

Of course, don't think that you can never snack. Who doesn't enjoy some popcorn at a movie or a dessert at a birthday celebration? But if something other than hunger seems to trigger all, or almost all, of your eating, reevaluate the way in which you feed your body.

Getting the Right Mix of Nutrients

Carbohydrates, proteins, and fats in your diet work together to provide energy and fuel for your body. The best approach to good nutrition is to eat some foods belonging to each of these categories at each meal.

Carbohydrates

Carbohydrates are one of your body's primary sources of energy and include fiber, starch, and sugar. You can divide them into complex carbs and simple carbs.

Complex carbohydrates

Complex carbohydrates are high in fiber and digest more slowly than simple carbohydrates, which makes them more filling. Complex carbs consist of sugar molecules that are strung together in long, complex chains. Complex carbs pack in more nutrients than simple carbs.

Eating complex carbs (versus simple carbs) can help you maintain a healthy weight and can help guard against type 2 diabetes and cardiovascular problems. They include fruits, vegetables, and whole grains:

>> **Fresh fruits and vegetables:** Healthier than canned or processed varieties because the fresh versions have more fiber and less sugar and salt than the others.

>> **Whole grain products:** Including flours, breads, and cereals, whole grain products provide better nutrition than refined or processed grains because a lot of the vitamins and fiber in grains are contained in the outer portion, which gets removed during processing.

People often call fiber *roughage* because the human digestive system can't effectively break down fibrous plant material. Fiber comes it two types:

>> **Soluble fiber:** Dissolves in water. Soluble fiber is in foods such as berries, oats, legumes, and potatoes. Soluble fiber passes slowly through your digestive system, helping you feel fuller longer.

>> **Insoluble fiber:** Fiber that your body can't break down or digest at all. Insoluble fiber helps prevent constipation, as well as aids in the movement of the partially undigested particles in your intestines that your body needs to eliminate.

TIP

You may feel intimidated by needing six servings of high fiber/complex carbohydrates per day, but you can really get those servings easily; fruits and vegetables, and whole grains can make up a large portion of needed fiber and carbohydrates.

Simple carbohydrates

You can find simple carbohydrates in sugary drinks, baked goods, desserts, breakfast cereals, milk, and many alcoholic beverages. Simple sugars can give you a quick burst of energy, and eating sugar or sugary products is the quickest way to raise your blood sugar if it drops too low. However, the energy burst doesn't last, and simple sugars don't do much for long-term performance.

Avoid simple sugars as much as you can because they raise your blood sugar levels and don't provide any long-term energy benefit. Persistently high sugar levels can put you at risk for type 2 diabetes, which many women are diagnosed with at midlife.

Proteins

Proteins are large, complex molecules that play an essential part in the structure, function, and regulation of all the cells and tissues in your body. Chains of small units called *amino acids*, which are linked together in certain sequences, make up protein.

Dietary sources of protein include

>> Meat, poultry, and fish

>> Eggs

>> Dairy products

>> Legumes (beans, lentils, chickpeas, and soybeans)

>> Nuts and seeds

Many foods that are high in protein also contain high levels of fat and cholesterol. By choosing lean cuts of meat and emphasizing the plant-based proteins in your diet, you can get adequate amounts of protein while staying as healthy as possible. Fish or chicken choices should be more frequent than red meat on your plate, and lower-fat dairy products can substitute for full-fat dairy.

Make proteins about 20 to 30 percent of your total daily calorie intake. Athletes may require a higher percentage of protein intake to support muscle recovery and growth.

Fats

Dietary fats are the fats that come from the food that you eat. The body breaks down dietary fats into parts called *fatty acids* that can then enter the bloodstream. The body can also make fatty acids from the carbohydrates in food.

Fatty acids have important roles in serving as energy for the muscles, heart, and other organs, as building blocks for cell membranes, and as energy storage for the body.

Besides providing the source for fatty acids, fats also

>> Help the body absorb certain (fat-soluble) vitamins, such as vitamin A, D, E, and K

>> Supply the body with more energy than carbohydrates or proteins

>> Contain almost twice as many calories as carbs and proteins

If someone needs to gain weight, high-fat foods can help. But those high-fat foods can also raise your cholesterol levels and increase your risk of heart disease, diabetes, and some cancers.

Not all dietary fats are the same. Different types of fats have different effects on the body. Some dietary fats are essential for bodily functions, some increase the risk for disease, and some help prevent disease. I discuss the two different general categories of fats in the following sections: saturated fats and unsaturated fats.

REMEMBER

Focus on eating more healthy fats (see the section "Unsaturated fats," later in this chapter) and limiting the unhealthier ones (discussed in the following section). Limit or eliminate processed foods that contain saturated trans-fat (and also more sugar, which I talk about in the section "Simple carbohydrates," earlier in this chapter).

Saturated fats

Saturated fats are usually solid at room temperature and mostly come from animal food products.

The Dietary Guidelines for Americans suggests that less than 10 percent of the calories that you take in during a day should come from saturated fats. The American Heart Association suggests a goal of no more than 6 percent per day.

Foods high in saturated fats include

>> Foods baked or fried in butter or margarine

>> Meats, including beef, lamb, pork, and poultry that includes the skin

>> Lard

>> Dairy products such as butter and cream

>> Whole milk and 2% milk

>> Whole-milk cheese or yogurt

>> Oils from coconuts, palm fruits, and palm kernels

Trans fats are a type of saturated fat created by adding hydrogen to vegetable oil, which causes the oil to become solid at room temperature. You can find trans fats in

>> Fried foods

>> Bakery goods

>> Hard margarines

>> Ice cream and other desserts

Saturated fats tend to raise levels of cholesterol in your blood. But there are two types of cholesterol (and saturated fats can raise the levels of both): LDL and HDL.

You may have heard low-density lipoprotein (LDL) referred to as the bad cholesterol. A high level of LDL in your bloodstream

>> Raises the risk for heart and blood vessel disease.

>> Can contribute to a condition called *atherosclerosis,* where plaques and fatty deposits build up in the inner walls of the arteries. This buildup of fat eventually blocks the blood flow to the heart and can lead to heart attacks.

Although saturated fats can also raise the level of high-density lipoprotein (HDL), called the good cholesterol, you may be able to raise your HDL levels without raising your LDL levels by eating beans, oily or fatty fish, and avocados.

Unsaturated fats

Unsaturated fats are fats that contain unsaturated fatty acid molecules. You can divide unsaturated fats into two broad categories: polyunsaturated and monosaturated.

POLYUNSATURATED FATS

Polyunsaturated fats usually come from plants or fish. The two categories of these fats are

>> **Omega-6 fatty acids:** Sources include corn oil, cottonseed oil, peanut oil, soybean oil, and sunflower oil. They lower your LDL (bad) cholesterol, but also lower your HDL (good) cholesterol.

>> **Omega-3 fatty acids:** Sources include salmon, anchovies, mackerel, herring, sardines, tuna, canola oil, soybean oil, flaxseed oil, soybeans, chia seeds, and walnuts. Diets high in Omega-3 fatty acids can lower the levels of *triglycerides* (fats) in your blood and may lower the risk of heart and blood vessel disease.

MONOUNSATURATED FATS

Monounsaturated fats contain fatty acids. These fats are found in many foods, including red meats and dairy products. However, red meat and dairy also have saturated fats (see the section "Saturated fats," earlier in this chapter), which you want to avoid.

Many plants and plant oils are high in monounsaturated fats but low in saturated fats. These include

>> Oils from olives, peanuts, canola seeds, safflower seeds, and sunflower seeds

>> Avocados

>> Pumpkin seeds

>> Nuts such as almonds, cashews, and pecans

>> Peanuts and peanut butter

WARNING

Depending on how the peanut butter is made, it can contain trans fats (see the section "Saturated fats," earlier in this chapter). To find healthier peanut butter options, look for peanut butters made with simply peanuts and salt, no trans fats.

Monounsaturated fats from plants may lower LDL (the bad cholesterol) and raise HDL (the good cholesterol). They may also help control blood sugar levels.

LOOKING FOR THE PERIMENOPAUSE DIET

I must apologize — I don't have a specific perimenopause diet to give you because one doesn't exist. Advertisers who try to sell you on a special or specific diet made just-for-women-in-perimenopause are leading you astray. You can certainly find healthy ways to eat in midlife, and if you're not already taking a good look at your eating habits and making some changes to accommodate the changes in your body, perimenopause provides a good time to reevaluate. But as far as a specific diet or a secret way to eat that magically works on women at this stage of life? Sorry, nope.

A healthy, mostly plant based diet that contains plenty of beneficial nutrients and fiber, staying well hydrated, as well as adding diversity to your diet, can help you move through perimenopause and into the next stage of your life more smoothly.

Keeping Your Bones Strong

Women in menopause are at risk of their bones getting thinner. Estrogen plays a large role in getting the calcium that's in your bloodstream into your bones, so when estrogen levels start to fluctuate and then decline, your bones are at risk. You may develop one of two conditions characterized by a decrease in mineral density and bone mass due to a lack of calcium in the body or an inability of the body to utilize that calcium:

>> **Osteopenia:** Bones are thinner and more fragile than healthy bones.

>> **Osteoporosis:** A more severe condition than osteopenia; bones are thin enough to put them at high risk of breaking.

Figure 13-1 shows a healthy bone and one that has osteoporosis, a condition characterized by the decrease in mineral density and bone mass.

Your bones don't begin to thin in menopause, and you don't necessarily have to lose bone density. Many lifestyle and dietary choices that you can make before menopause can protect your bones and help prevent osteoporosis and fractures (see Chapter 11 for a lot more on bones).

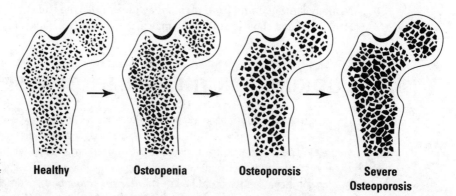

FIGURE 13-1:
The stages of osteoporosis.

| Healthy | Osteopenia | Osteoporosis | Severe Osteoporosis |

Diet and exercise give you two easy ways to improve the health of your bones.

To better understand osteoporosis, it helps to know how bones are built. Each bone contains cells that build bone (osteoblasts) and cells that break down and clear away bone (osteoclasts). They are like two crews — the builders and the removers — and they work in sync to remodel your bones. Osteoclasts remove bone by dissolving it. In the area where bone has been dissolved and cleared away, a small hole is left. Get enough of these holes, without refilling them with something to make the bones strong again, and you end up with weak bones that have a lot of holes — and hence, osteoporosis.

The bone-building osteoblasts need calcium to help fill the holes, and if you don't have enough calcium in your bloodstream, the holes remain. Bone building exceeds bone breakdown naturally for the first 30 years or so of your life. Around age 30, you reach your peak bone mass, which is the maximum amount of bone density that you'll ever have. After age 30, you have to do all that you can to keep the holes from getting larger; you need to make sure you get enough calcium, as well as other vitamins, to allow the building crew to keep working.

About 25 million Americans have osteoporosis, and most of them are women. If you take action in perimenopause, then you can prevent the disease. And if you find yourself diagnosed in your perimenopausal years with osteoporosis, you have treatments available. A fracture, especially a hip fracture, can change the quality of the rest of your life, and 50 percent of women who suffer a hip fracture never return to their former level of function.

The following sections describe essentials to include in your diet in order to keep your bones healthy and strong.

Calcium

Calcium is an important player in the bone-building story. Your body needs calcium to build new bone and to keep every cell in your body functioning. Under age 50, women need about 1,000 milligrams (mg) of calcium per day to keep up the bone-building process, and after age 50, it increases to 1,200 mg per day.

Many foods are naturally high in calcium (see Chapter 11 for a list of how much calcium is typically found in foods you eat every day). Calcium occurs naturally in

>> Dairy products

>> Green leafy vegetables, such as kale and collard greens

>> Fish that include bones

>> Tofu

>> Almonds

And certain juices, non-dairy milks, and breads are *calcium fortified,* meaning the production process includes adding calcium to the food or drink.

Become a label reader, and then it becomes a simple math equation: Add up the amount of calcium that's in all the foods that you consume in a day, and then supplement whatever you find missing to get you to that 1,000 or 1,200 mg recommended age-based daily dose. Your body can easily absorb the supplements calcium citrate and calcium carbonate, but try to get at least half of your needed calcium from your dietary intake because foods naturally contain a variety of nutrients that work together to support bone-health. Calcium from food sources is typically easier for your body to digest and absorb compared to calcium supplements. Excess calcium intake from supplements can lead to constipation and the formation of kidney stones. Some antacids, such as Tums, have 500 mg of calcium in them; easy to tolerate and good for gas problems, too!

Findings from the Women's Health Initiative study show that women who take calcium every day have 29 percent fewer hip fractures than those who don't. Many foods now available have been enriched with calcium; you just need to read those labels!

Vitamin D

Your body needs vitamin D to properly absorb calcium. Low blood levels of vitamin D may relate to a host of other chronic health problems, such as diabetes, inflammatory bowel disease, and certain cancers. But both the studies and recommended daily doses of vitamin D are controversial. Based on the bone benefits alone, women under age 70 should take 600 to 800 international units (IUs) of vitamin D3 daily, and for women over 70, at least 800 IUs daily. The upper limit of safe intake is 4,000 IUs daily, depending on individual chronic illnesses and known blood levels of vitamin D.

The American Association of Clinical Endocrinologists states that when checking blood levels of vitamin D, values between 30 and 50 nanograms per milliliter (ng/mL) have bone health benefits (as well as other benefits, such as better immune function and a positive impact on moods). Some doctors check your vitamin D levels by using a blood test to see whether you need to supplement with higher doses of vitamin D3. Most healthy adults who don't have symptoms of vitamin D deficiency (fatigue, loss of appetite, muscle weakness, bone pain, or hair loss) don't need to have their vitamin D blood levels checked.

Certain medical conditions may interfere with your body's absorption of vitamin D:

» Weight loss (bariatric) surgery

» Taking anti-seizure medication to treat epilepsy

» Taking steroids to treat an inflammatory condition

If you fall into one of the groups in the preceding list, your doctor probably checks your vitamin D level periodically and has you supplement as needed.

You can get vitamin D from about 15 minutes of daily sun exposure because the UV rays in sunshine stimulate the skin to produce vitamin D. However, sunscreens (UV blockers) can blunt the ability of the sun's UV rays to trigger the production of vitamin D. (But don't use this as an excuse to not use sunscreen!)

Vitamin K, potassium, and magnesium

Vitamin K, potassium, and magnesium all help in the bone-building journey. Here's a list of which foods provide these essential nutrients:

>> **Vitamin K:** Collard greens, turnip greens, broccoli, soybeans, carrots, edamame, pumpkin, and pomegranates

>> **Potassium:** Sweet potatoes, white potatoes, tomato sauce, watermelon, bananas, spinach, beets, black beans, and white beans

>> **Magnesium:** Spinach, dark chocolate, avocado, pumpkin seeds, cashews, bananas, beans, and tofu

Managing Weight

Fortunately, or unfortunately, you don't have to crack a code or work out a magic trick to keep weight off in perimenopause. Hormone therapy by itself doesn't cause weight loss, and any advertising or sales pitch that tells you it will rev up your metabolism is selling you a false bill of goods.

Avoiding the insidious weight creep

Many studies have looked at weight and metabolism in perimenopause and menopause, and none have concluded that perimenopause causes metabolic changes that are major enough to cause changes in weight separate from the changes that occur from aging alone.

If your perimenopausal transition takes five to six years until you reach menopause, you might certainly gain 1 to 2 pounds per year, resulting in an 8- to 14-pound weight gain over that period.

During perimenopause, several factors can lead to weight gain:

>> If you're less active than when you were younger, you tend to lose muscle, as well as not burning off those calories.

>> Weight that accumulates during perimenopause tends to revolve around your midsection, called *abdominal deposition of fat* — and this type of fat can lead to cardiovascular problems.

If the pattern of gaining more weight every year continues, then by the time you reach menopause, you might think the hormones are to blame when, not so suddenly, you have to deal with medical conditions, high cholesterol, and possibly even obesity.

However you do it, you need to establish a *calorie deficit,* meaning you must eat fewer calories than you burn off through activity. Make your meals, and all eating, thoughtful and planned.

REMEMBER

Weight loss doesn't depend on balancing hormones. You need to establish and follow a food and lifestyle plan that can serve you for the rest of your life. Being consistent, listening to your hunger cues, and having a basic knowledge of nutrition can go a long way to living your nutritionally healthiest and best life.

Following basic eating rules

Really, no single diet works for everyone, or for everyone in perimenopause. Eating a lower-carb, higher-protein, plant-based, or Mediterranean diet doesn't guarantee that you lose weight, keep it off, and have a healthier life. Whichever type of eating plan you decide works for you just needs to follow some basic rules:

>> Eat nutrient-dense, balanced meals, including

• Many fresh seasonal vegetables and fruits

• Lean protein, including protein from plants (discussed in the section "Proteins," earlier in this chapter)

• Whole grain carbs (flip to the section "Carbohydrates," earlier in this chapter, for details on the good carbs)

• Dairy (if you can tolerate it and if that is something that you desire to include in your diet)

• Healthy fats (see the section "Unsaturated fats," earlier in this chapter)

>> Practice mindful, distraction-free eating at a table (not at your desk or standing by the fridge) and plan your meals.

>> Limit your alcohol intake, and limit or eliminate processed and packaged foods that contain long lists of ingredients because processed foods are stripped of essential nutrients and are often high in sugar, salt, and unhealthy fats.

>> Try not to eat to manage emotions. Get professional help for disordered eating, binge eating, or extreme dieting habits. Flip back to the section "Identifying social and emotional eating," earlier in this chapter, for more information.

>> Don't follow extreme or restrictive diets that eliminate entire food groups or create a fear of food. You can and should enjoy eating.

IS MEDICATION FOR WEIGHT LOSS SAFE, AND DOES IT WORK?

At the time I'm writing this book, it seems that healthcare providers are increasingly prescribing various medications to treat obesity and help with weight loss. The medical profession has begun to look at people who are overweight and obese as suffering from a chronic metabolic medical condition, rather than perpetuating the misconception that more willpower is the solution for weight loss. You can now find several prescription medications available to help people lose up to 15 percent of their body weight or more over time, with the goal of better health and fewer chronic medical conditions like diabetes and heart disease.

These medications have actually been around for decades. They work on receptors in various parts of your body to send the brain a message that you're full. They also slow down food's *transit time* through your system (the amount of time it takes for food to pass through your stomach and intestines), which means you feel fuller for longer.

Much controversy exists about who should be on these medications, and the medications come with many potential side effects. Sometimes, patients have to take these medications for years — or risk gaining weight back after discontinuing them.

If you think that you may want to use one of these medications for weight loss, have a conversation with your healthcare provider. You can see whether you're a candidate based on your individual circumstances, your family history, and your goals and expectations. Always work with a registered dietitian or nutritional counselor while on the medication to make sure that your dietary habits provide adequate nutrition and that you're losing weight in the safest and healthiest way possible.

Chapter **14**

Getting into an Exercise Plan Before Menopause

You can find so many reasons to make exercising a primary part of your life at any age, but especially during your perimenopausal life, while you prepare for the transition to menopause.

In this chapter, you will see how regular exercise can provide tremendous health benefits. Exercise is an important part of a healthy lifestyle. In perimenopause it is so important to adopt lifestyle habits that will make the transition to menopause easier, and exercise helps reduce stress, improves flexibility and balance, and keeps the heart and bones strong.

Benefiting from Exercise

Exercise is vital to your health and well-being. The single best thing that you can do to stay healthy, live longer, and prepare yourself for menopause is to keep moving.

The following sections discuss some of the many ways exercise can serve you in perimenopause and beyond.

Mental health

Exercising regularly can significantly support good mental health. You may see this as a vital asset while fluctuating hormones in perimenopause add to mood problems that may have already been present (see Chapter 9 for more on perimenopause's effect on your mental health).

Engaging in physical activity can enhance the production of *endorphins*, hormones that help to elevate mood, reduce stress, and promote a sense of well-being. (You can read about hormones in Chapter 6.) Regular exercise and a nutritious diet (see Chapter 13) can also help reduce levels of stress hormones.

Physical activity can also act as a distraction, allowing you to temporarily shift focus away from daily worries and stressors, while boosting your energy levels.

Also, engaging in regular exercise can lead to improvements in overall body image and self-esteem. Making sustainable life-long lifestyle changes can help promote a sense of confidence and accomplishment.

Brain function

Exercise increases blood flow to the brain, which can help improve memory, concentration, and mental clarity. Exercise has been shown to enhance memory and cognitive function. It can improve both short-term and long-term memory. Exercise promotes something called *neuroplasticity,* which is the brain's ability to reorganize and adapt. This can support learning and skill development. Regular exercise can improve attention span and the ability to concentrate on tasks.

Energy and sleep

Being physically active can contribute to better quality of sleep. Regular exercise can help regulate sleep patterns, while a balanced diet (discussed in Chapter 13) can provide the essential nutrients to support healthy sleep cycles.

Besides getting a good night's sleep, exercising can help you combat fatigue and can have a dramatic (positive!) effect on your energy levels.

Making Exercise a Regular Habit

REMEMBER

Although you may need to check with your doctor before you start an exercise program — especially if you have health concerns or haven't exercised in a long time — this chapter provides some basic pieces of advice about exercising in perimenopause and menopause. It's important to note that the effects of exercise on health and overall well-being will vary from person to person and depend on the type, intensity and duration of exercise. Consistency is key, so incorporating regular physical activity into your routine is a good way to benefit from an exercise routine over the long term.

Setting Midlife Exercise Goals

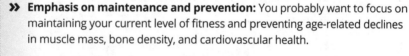

Whether you have a long history of marathon running or have never been a big fan of working out, the role that fitness plays in your life — the how, why, and when of your fitness habits — changes while you age. Your physical ability changes while your body ages, as does your risk of injury. Before setting your fitness routine, or adapting your current one, reassess what you want to get out of your workout routine, and keep in mind that fitness goals for women over 40 may be slightly different from the goals of earlier years (whether you wanted that bikini-ready body or to crush your competition on the basketball court back in the day).

Here are some ways that your fitness goals may change when you enter middle age:

WARNING

>> **Emphasis on maintenance and prevention:** You probably want to focus on maintaining your current level of fitness and preventing age-related declines in muscle mass, bone density, and cardiovascular health.

According to the American Council on Exercise, sedentary adults between the ages of 30 and 80 can experience as much as 40 percent loss of their muscular strength because of reduced muscle mass.

>> **Injury prevention and joint health:** The best exercises support joint health and injury reduction, focusing more on flexibility, balance, and stability training.

>> **Bone health and osteoporosis prevention:** Weight-bearing exercises and resistance training are excellent for bone health.

>> **Metabolism and weight management:** As metabolism naturally slows down with age, exercise goals may in part focus on healthy body weight.

>> **Functional fitness for an active, independent life:** These are exercises that enhance your ability to perform everyday tasks, such as lifting, carrying, bending, and climbing stairs.

>> **Heart health and cardiovascular fitness:** You may focus on cardiovascular exercises to maintain heart health and reduce the risk of cardiovascular diseases that become more prevalent with age.

>> **Flexibility and range of motion:** Maintaining flexibility and range of motion supports joint health, prevents stiffness, and maintains mobility.

>> **Mind-body connection and stress management:** Practices such as yoga and tai chi, which promote the mind-body connection and emphasize stress reduction, may become more integral to an exercise routine in midlife.

>> **Social and community engagement:** Exercise activities provide excellent opportunities for social interaction and community engagement, both of which improve a person's overall well-being (and make exercise more fun).

Looking after your body and mind

Many different types of physical activity can help protect the heart, strengthen the bones and muscles, and maintain and improve balance, body weight, mood, and a general sense of well-being.

You can include a variety of exercises a few times a week (ideally five or more days a week) to keep the routine fun and interesting. Consider

>> Aerobics, in classes or individually

>> Biking or spinning

>> Brisk walking

>> Dancing

>> Interval training

>> Jogging

>> Tennis

>> Weight training

Incorporating weight and strength training

After age 30, you begin to lose about 1 percent of your muscle mass every year. Because muscle burns fat, this muscle reduction leads to fat-based weight gain.

You can reverse this trend by using these types of exercise routines (and flip to the section "Getting Pumped with Strength Training Exercises," later in this chapter, for some suggested exercises):

>> **Weight training:** Here's where you work the major muscle groups, including your legs, arms, butt and core, by using some basic moves with weights, such as free weights or gym equipment.

>> **Strength training:** Also called *resistance training,* you can do these exercises with your body weight alone, using elastic or stretchy tubing. You can go to your local gym to do strength training, but you can find entire resistance-training programs that you can do in your home without any equipment.

Stretching those muscles

Do some stretching every day, especially if you typically sit most of the day. Muscles in the back of your legs, as well as in your back and neck, tend to stiffen up when they're not used, so to stay flexible, you need to do some stretching. Practicing mindful stretches can help you in a variety of ways:

>> Make your muscles and connective tissue more flexible

>> Help your nervous system by promoting relaxation and reducing pain

>> Improve sleep quality

>> Help lessen depressive symptoms

Also, incorporating stretching before and after physical activity can better prepare the body for a strong workout and help it cool down after one.

You can find so many ways to stretch that entire books have been written about this topic — including *Stretching For Dummies,* by LeReine Chabut (Wiley). Proper stretching increases your flexibility and your range of motion.

Here are the basics of stretching:

>> Aim for stretching each muscle group for about 30 seconds.

>> Stretching should feel slightly uncomfortable, but not painful.

>> Use a strap or a towel to help you stretch, if you need one.

>> Don't bounce when you stretch because this puts sudden uncontrolled force on your muscles and tendons, increasing the risk of strains, pulls, and even tears.

>> Progress through your stretching: Go from a comfortable stretch to relaxing into the stretch, to deeply stretching those muscles.

>> Remember to breathe.

Keeping Yourself on Balance

Balance often worsens with age. Poor balance can cause problems while you get older because it can increase the risk of falls and fractures. Any activity that strengthens your legs and core can help with balance.

Yoga and tai chi include postures and positions that specifically focus on balance. Balance exercises that you can do at home include

>> Standing on one foot, first with eyes open and then closed

>> Heel-to-toe walking (like a sobriety test)

>> Walking lunges

>> Sitting on a balance ball while using upper-body weights

Looking at Workout Intensity

Whether you're doing cardiovascular exercise, such as running, or resistance training (and you should be doing both), determine the intensity with which to do those activities, both in terms of duration and as it relates to your heart rate.

Beginners: If you're new to exercise and may have low fitness levels, start with shorter sessions of about 15-20 minutes, three days a week. Focus on building endurance gradually to avoid overexertion or injury. Briskly walking or hiking on low hills can be low intensity cardiovascular exercises if you keep an eye on your level of comfort while active. You should be able to continue to breathe normally and even carry on a conversation while at a low intensity of exercise.

For general fitness: For overall cardiovascular fitness, aim for 150 minutes of moderate intensity aerobic exercise (running, dancing, hiking, jogging, aerobic classes, biking) spread over 3-5 days. As your fitness increases, you can increase the intensity of the exercise (where you are working hard, and sweating, *NOT* having a conversation.) The ideal goal should be about 30-40 minutes of moderate intensity exercise most days of the week.

Sets and reps

The number of repetitions (reps) and sets of an exercise routine that you do depends on your fitness goals: If you do high reps with lighter weights you will build muscular endurance, and if you do heavier weights with fewer reps you will bulk up the muscles. The American College of Sports medicine has the following recommendations:

>> **To build strength:** Do fewer repetitions per set: 8 to 12 reps and 2 to 6 sets per session. Take a 1- to 3-minute rest in between.

>> **To boost muscular endurance:** Complete sets of 10 to 25 reps with a 30- to 60-second rest in between the sets.

TIP

The best workout routines for women over 40 are those that you can change up regularly. Avoid doing the exact same workout day after day because changing up the routine avoids boredom and reduces overuse injuries. Instead, do a variety of exercises which target different muscle groups to promote more well-rounded fitness.

You can choose from many workout routines that you can do regularly without taking too much time out of your day. Ease into these exercise routines to avoid injury; start with something simple, such as walking. A basic walking routine begins with an easy warm-up; a few minutes of slow, easy walking to warm up your muscles. Then start to pick up the pace and begin to take a quick stroll around your neighborhood. Choose a comfortable pace, initially for a short duration of 15 minutes. As your fitness improves, pick up the pace and increase the duration, paying attention to form: keeping shoulders relaxed, back straight, and eventually adding some light hand weights to the routine.

Using heart rate to choose an exercise option

Your heart rate provides a real-time indicator of how hard your heart is working during your exercise. It helps you gauge the intensity of your workout.

>> **Low intensity:** Spend at least 20 minutes at 60 percent of your maximum heart rate (see the sidebar "Using a heart rate monitor," in this chapter, for info about keeping tabs on your ticker). Low-intensity exercises can include

- Yoga

- Pilates

- Mobility and flexibility exercises

- Walking at a speed of 2 to 3 miles per hour

» **Moderate intensity:** Spend at least 20 to 30 minutes at 70 percent of your maximum heart rate. Good moderate-intensity exercises include

- Brisk walking or jogging
- Playing tennis
- Using an elliptical trainer
- Bicycling on level ground
- Water aerobics
- Swimming
- Dancing

» **High intensity:** Spend at least 25 to 40 minutes at 80 percent of your maximum heart rate. Good choices for high-intensity workouts include

- Running.
- Cycling at a rate faster than 10 miles per hour.
- Lap swimming.
- Plyometrics (also called *jump training*).
- Explosive training (which combines speed, strength, and power training). This involves dynamic movements that require rapid and forceful muscle contractions.

USING A HEART RATE MONITOR

If you use a heart rate monitor, you can have instant access to your heart rate. Knowing your heart rate at any given moment gives you a great way to figure out whether you should push harder in your workout routine or need to back down a little. Knowing how hard you must exercise (and how hard you are exercising) can help you to reach your goals more quickly.

Here's an explanation of heart measurements:

- **Resting heart rate:** The number of beats per minute (bpm) that your heart beats when you're completely at rest. It's the lowest rate your heart will normally beat because it occurs when you're not being active. Take your resting heart rate when you're sitting or lying down, and you don't have anything stimulating your heart (such as caffeine, illness, or stress). A normal resting heart rate falls between 60 and 100 bpm.

- **Maximum heart rate:** As fast as your heart can beat. To calculate a very broad estimate of your maximum heart rate, subtract your age from 220. (For example, if you're 40, your maximum heart rate is 220 – 40, or 180 bpm.)

- **Target heart rate:** A goal of how fast you want your heart to beat while you exercise. A low-intensity workout should get your heart rate to about 60 percent of your maximum heart rate (so if your maximum heart rate is 180 bpm, aim for 108 bpm). For moderate intensity exercise, get your heart rate at 70 percent of your maximum (126 bpm in my example). And get your heart up to 80 percent of your maximum heart rate (144 bpm) for a high-intensity workout.

You can get different fitness benefits by exercising in different heart rate zones. Working out in different heart rate zones offers various fitness benefits because it allows you to target specific aspects of your fitness and achieve different training objectives. Here are the key fitness benefits associated with working out in different heart rate zones:

ZONE 1-Recovery zone (50-60% of maximum heart rate) benefits: Training in this zone helps endurance, aerobic endurance, improves overall cardiovascular health, and aids in recovery. It is ideal for beginners and active recovery days.

ZONE 2-Aerobic zone (60-70% of maximum heart rate) benefits: Training in this zone further develops aerobic endurance, enhances fat utilization for energy, and increases stamina.

ZONE 3-Aerobic threshold zone (70-80% of maximum heart rate) benefits: This zone improves aerobic capacity, increases the ability to sustain higher intensity efforts, and enhances cardiovascular fitness.

ZONE 4-Anaerobic threshold zone (80-90% of maximum heart rate) benefits: Training in this zone improves speed, power, and race performance. It allows you to sustain higher intensity of exercise for longer periods.

ZONE 5-Maximal effort zone (90-100% of maximum heart rate) benefits: This zone should be used sparingly due to its intensity. It is usually reserved for elite athletes who need to improve their maximal power output and sprinting capabilities.

By incorporating workouts in different heart rate zones, you can create a well-rounded training program that targets various aspects of fitness. Consider consulting with a trainer or other fitness professional to help monitor your heart rate and set goals for maximum safety and fitness.

Getting Pumped with Strength Training Exercises

The following sections provide some simple but effective exercises that you can do to keep your muscles strong and your body flexible and healthy. These exercises provide a variety of easy to do strength and resistance exercises for an overall body workout. They can help you preserve muscle mass and keep your bones strong.

The benefits of strength training in perimenopause don't include big biceps or washboard abs. This type of training can help you maintain a strong and healthy body that's less prone to illness. Building and maintaining lean muscle mass can increase your resting metabolic rate, improve joint stability, and help improve balance.

TIP

When you do resistance training by using elastic bands, dumbbells, or your own body weight, do enough repetitions so that you feel comfortably fatigued after 10 to 12 repetitions (reps). Repeat 3 sets of reps during your workout.

Forearm plank

The forearm plank (see Figure 14-1) can improve your posture, as well as strengthening your core, arms, shoulders, and legs. Just follow these steps:

1. **Begin by lying on the floor with your forearms flat on the floor.**

   Align your elbows directly under your shoulders.

2. **Engage your core and raise your body off the floor.**

   Keep you forearms on the floor and your body in a straight line from head to foot.

   Keep your abdominals engaged, and don't let your hips rise or fall.

3. **Hold this pose for 30 seconds.**

   Place your knees on the ground if keeping the straight line becomes painful or difficult.

4. **Relax your body back into your position in Step 1.**

5. **Repeat Steps 2 through 4 until you complete the reps that you want to do.**

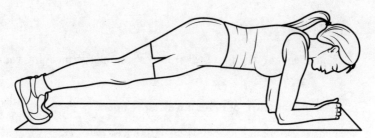

FIGURE 14-1:
The forearm
plank.

Modified pushup

To do a modified pushup (see Figure 14-2) — which can strengthen your core, shoulders, and arms — follow these steps:

1. **Begin in the kneeling position on a mat.**

   Have your hands positioned directly below your shoulders, your knees behind your hips, and your back long and angled.

2. **Tighten your abdominals and bend your elbows to lower your chest towards the floor.**

   Keep your gaze in front of you.

3. **Press your chest back up to the starting position in Step 1.**

4. **Repeat Steps 2 and 3 for your designated number of reps.**

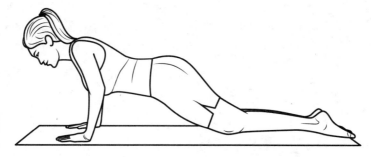

FIGURE 14-2:
The modified
pushup.

Basic squat

The basic squat (see Figure 14-3) works your *glutes* (meaning your rear) and legs. Follow these steps:

1. **Stand tall with your feet hip-distance apart.**

   Have your hips, knees, and toes all facing forward.

2. **Bend your knees and extend your butt backward.**

   Act like you're about to sit in a chair.

3. **Keep your knees behind your toes and put your weight on your heels.**

   Once you get to the position of the squat, return to standing up fully — there is no time maintaining the squat position.

4. **Rise back up to a standing position.**

5. **Repeat Steps 2 through 4 enough times to get your reps in.**

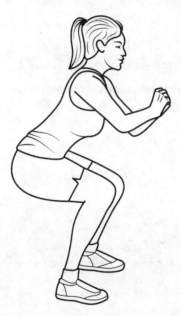

FIGURE 14-3:
The basic squat.

Chest fly

Follow these steps to perform the chest fly (see Figure 14-4), which helps strengthen your chest, shoulder, and arm muscles:

1. **Lie down on a firm surface.**

   You can use a bench or lie on a mat on the floor.

2. **Hold a pair of light dumbbells close to your chest with your elbows bent at 90-degree angles.**

3. **Raise the dumbbells above your chest, palms facing each other.**

4. **Straighten your elbows all the way.**

   But don't lock your elbows because you can *hyperextend* your elbow joint, opening it beyond the normal, healthy range of motion. Hyperextension causes ligament and cartilage damage over time.

WARNING

5. **Slowly lower your arms out to the sides, maintaining a slight bend in the elbow, until your elbows are at chest level.**

6. **Repeat Steps 3 through 5 for your designated number of reps.**

Shoulder overhead press

You can do the shoulder overhead press exercise (which works your chest, shoulders, arms, and upper back) while either standing or sitting. See Figure 14-5. Follow these steps:

1. **Start with your feet hip distance apart on the floor (either sitting or standing).**

2. **Bring your elbows out to the sides of your body and position your arms so that dumbbells are at either side of your head.**

3. **Raise the dumbbells up until your arm is fully extended.**

   Keep your abdominals tight and elbows straight.

4. **Slowly return your arms to the position in Step 2.**

   Control the descent of your arms to put those muscles through their paces.

5. **Repeat Steps 3 and 4 until you complete the number of reps in your set.**

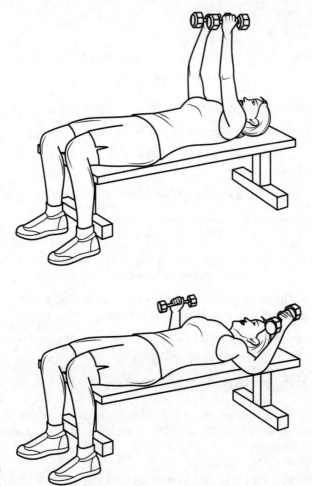

FIGURE 14-4:
The chest fly.

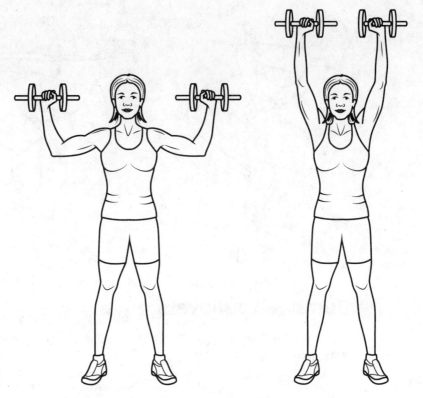

FIGURE 14-5:
The standard
overhead press.

Triceps kickback

Follow these steps to do a triceps kickback (see Figure 14-6), which (okay, obviously) strengthens your *triceps*, the muscles on the back of your upper arms:

1. Stand slightly bent forward, knees shoulder width apart.

2. Bend your elbows at a 90-degree angle.

3. Slowly straighten your arm backwards.

4. Just as slowly return your arm to the 90-degree-angle position in Step 2.

5. Repeat Steps 3 and 4 for the number of reps that you want to do.

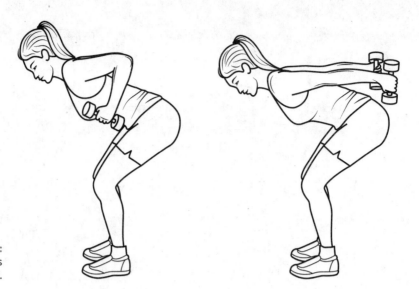

FIGURE 14-6:
The triceps
kickback.

Dumbbell pullovers

To do a dumbbell pullover (see Figure 14-7), which can strengthen your chest and arms, follow these steps:

1. **Lie down on a bench so that your back, neck, and head are fully supported.**

2. **Position your arms extended over your head, at the same level as your head, not lower**

3. **Extend your arms toward the ceiling, over your chest.**

   Keep a strong back and core, and have your palms facing each other, with your elbows slightly bent.

4. **Extend the weights back over your head.**

   Take 3 or 4 seconds to return the weights from over your chest to the position in Step 2.

5. **Repeat Steps 3 and 4 until you complete your set of reps.**

Side leg lifts

You can get your core, glutes, lower back, and legs into shape by doing side leg lifts (see Figure 14-8). Just follow these steps:

1. **Lie on your side on a firm but comfortable surface.**

   Use something like a mat on the floor.

2. **Keep your body, from your shoulders to your feet, in a straight line.**

3. **Engage your core, and slowly lift the upper leg straight up in the air.**

   Don't swing the leg.

4. **Return your leg to the ground slowly.**

5. **Repeat Steps 3 and 4 until you complete all your reps.**

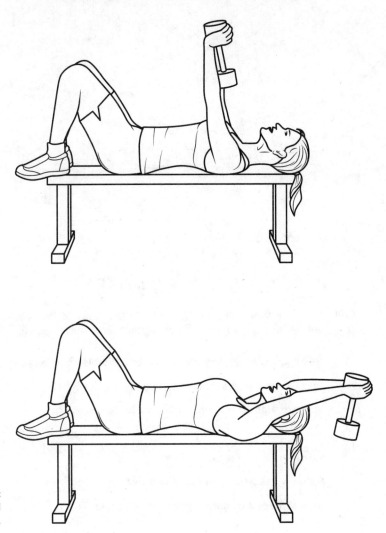

FIGURE 14-7:
The dumbbell
pullover.

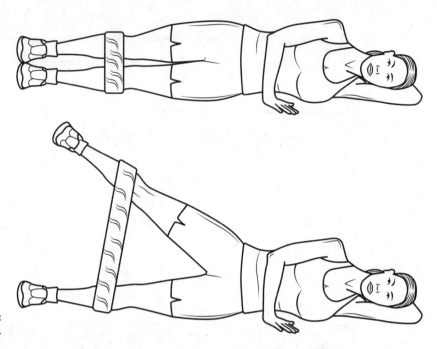

FIGURE 14-8:
Side leg lifts.

TIP

You can also do this exercise using an elastic leg band to add tension and make the workout more intense.

Single leg hamstring bridge

The single leg hamstring bridge (see Figure 14-9) helps strengthen your lower back, glutes, and legs. To do this exercise, follow these steps:

1. Lie on your back with your knees bent, hip-distance apart.

2. Squeeze your *glutes* (butt muscles).

3. Lift your hips off the mat and into a bridge position.

4. Straighten one leg slowly.

5. Slowly bring that leg back down.

6. Follow Steps 2 through 5 for the other leg.

7. Repeat Steps 2 through 6 to get your reps in.

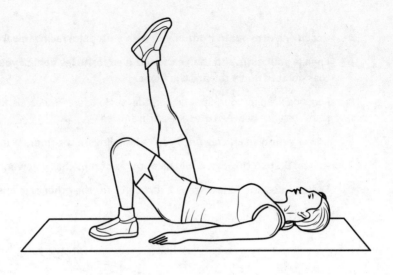

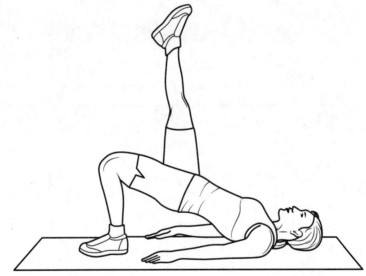

FIGURE 14-9:
Single leg
hamstring bridge.

Bird dog

Follow these steps to do the bird dog (see Figure 14-10), which can help you hone your core:

1. **Kneel on all fours on a mat.** Your hands should be directly under your shoulders and knees should be under your hips.

   Engage your core muscles by drawing your navel up toward your spine.

2. **Reach one arm out in front of you with your palm facing inward.**

3. **Engage your core, and then extend the opposite leg behind you, keeping toes pointed down toward the floor.**

   Focus on keeping your hips and pelvis level. Hold for 3-5 seconds, keeping a stable balance between the raised arm and leg.

4. **Lower your arm and leg until you're kneeling on the floor, as in Step 1.**

5. **Repeat Steps 2 through 4 for the number of reps that you want to do.**

6. **Switch sides and follow Steps 2 through 5 for the other arm and leg.**

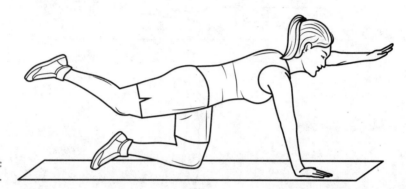

FIGURE 14-10:
The bird dog.

Chapter 15

Understanding and Preventing Bone Loss

You've probably seen that old TV commercial that starts with an elderly lady on the floor groaning, "I've fallen, and I can't get up!" Maybe you looked at that woman and said, "That's terrible — but that will never be me." You also may know someone who fell and fractured a bone — a hip, ankle, a wrist — and somehow their life has never been the same since. How can you keep that from happening to you?

It's a fact that our bones get weaker while we move toward menopause, making them more susceptible to breaking. But you can do a variety of things to keep your bones from getting so thin that a step-down off a curb in the wrong way, or a trip over a loosely placed rug, would result in a fracture that you may have difficulty recovering from.

Bone loss is progressive. It gets worse with age, worse with decreasing hormone levels, and much worse with a lack of exercise and a poor diet. You can mitigate the effects of bone loss by managing your risk factors in perimenopause before the bone loss becomes severe.

During perimenopause, really consider your bones and start doing everything that you need to do to keep them strong. In this chapter, you can find out about bone health, how bone loss occurs, and steps that you can take to decrease the chance that osteoporosis and fractures may happen to you.

Bone Building, Growth, and Remodeling

Bones are filled with cells that are considered bone builders (called *osteoblasts*) and cells that clear away bone (*osteoclasts*). The process of building new bone and removing or clearing away old bone is called *remodeling* and takes place throughout your life.

Over time, bone breaks down, and new bone replaces it:

>> **Osteoclasts:** When old bone dissolves, it creates a cavity in the bone, and osteoclasts essentially recycle the cleared-away bone cells, sending them into the bloodstream, where the body's organs can use the minerals (such as calcium and phosphorus) that are removed from the bone to perform their functions.

>> **Osteoblasts:** These cells build new bone and try to close up the cavities in the bones to provide new strength and new density to the bone.

In children, bones are continually growing longer and denser. The denser the bones are, the harder it is to break them. Although peak bone growth usually happens in the teenage years, peak bone density occurs around age 30. At this age, your body replaces as much bone as it loses. But starting at around age 40, your body replaces less bone that is lost, which causes the bones to become thinner and weaker.

Two conditions can occur when you start to lose bone density:

>> **Osteopenia:** A condition in which your bones are weaker than they should be, but not yet to the extent where you're at serious risk of injury

>> **Osteoporosis:** A much more severe condition that progresses from osteopenia, in which a simple fall may cause your bones to break

You may observe in your menopausal friends and relatives who have osteoporosis these signs. They may

>> Appear shorter than they used to

>> Have a noticeable hump on their back

>> Bend forward when they try to stand up straight, unable to stand fully upright

>> Fall and fracture a wrist or a hip

Figure 15-1 shows a spectrum of bone densities.

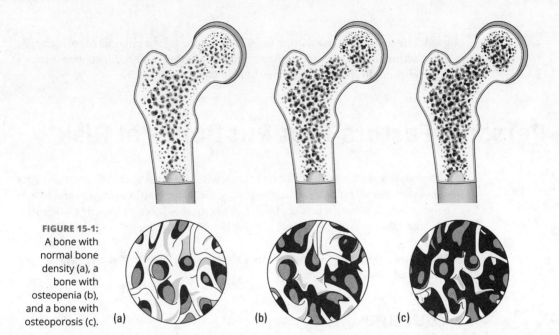

FIGURE 15-1: A bone with normal bone density (a), a bone with osteopenia (b), and a bone with osteoporosis (c).

(a) (b) (c)

TIP

If you start building strong and dense bones when you're young, the loss of bone density that starts to happen at midlife causes fewer problems for you. The higher your peak bone density, the better chance you have of keeping your bones healthy.

Regulating Bones with Hormones

Hormones affect the amount and the speed of bone remodeling and rebuilding; they play a part in your risk for osteoporosis and fracture. Estrogen, specifically, regulates bone metabolism, so you need it to maintain bone health.

Perimenopause is a time of fluctuating levels of estrogen, and the amount of estrogen made during this time may vary widely. Estrogen promotes the activity of *osteoblasts*, the cells that make new bone. When estrogen levels are low, osteoblasts make too little new bone, so bones have a harder time maintaining their structure.

At midlife, the bone destruction cells (*osteoclasts*) are starting to work faster than the bone-builders, so perimenopause is a perfect time to help the bone-building cells try to work more efficiently.

You don't have to wait until you enter menopause to address the bone loss that will ultimately occur because of low estrogen levels. Perimenopause gives you a good time to focus on preventing bone loss, to lessen your chances of osteoporosis and fracture later on. Decide with your doctor whether your perimenopause treatment plan might include hormones to help with bone health.

Personal Factors That Put Bones at Risk

Although you reached your full height somewhere around your 15th birthday, your bones continue to remodel throughout your life: They continue to gain and to lose bone in cycles. Some factors that you can't control — such as genetics, body size, age, and family history — can affect this bone remodeling process.

The following sections discuss some factors that influence the strength of your bones while you grow older.

Your age

Because bone-building cells don't work as efficiently after age 40, anyone over the age of 40 is at risk for thinning bones. After age 50, osteoporosis affects about 20 percent of women (meaning one in five), so the age from 40 to 50 is a critical time period for bone density awareness. Don't find yourself in that category of women who find out they had osteoporosis only after they break a bone! Do all that you can to keep your bones strong and prevent osteoporosis while you're still in perimenopause.

Family history

If you don't know about your family history when it comes to bone density, fractures, and osteoporosis, ask and investigate. Is your mom 2 inches shorter than she used to be? Is your older sister a little bent over when she walks? A family history of osteoporosis and fractures gives you important information about your personal risk factors that you can discuss with your healthcare provider.

Studies show that these are significant risks factors for the occurrence of osteoporosis:

>> Close relatives who have osteoporosis, especially your mother

>> Previous fractures in family members

You can't change your family history, but having information about family members can prompt you and your doctor toward earlier testing, intervention, and treatment in the perimenopausal period to get a jump start on maintaining bone health and strength beyond your midlife years.

Your ethnicity

In taking into consideration all the many risk factors that can contribute to bone loss, consider whether your ethnicity can add to that risk. Bone mineral density and fracture rates vary among women of differing ethnicities:

» **Bone mineral density (BMD):** Most reports suggest that BMD is highest in African American women.

» **Osteoporosis and low bone density:** Most common in white women, and next most common in Asian women.

» **Fracture rates:** White women have the highest fracture rates.

Researchers don't know why different ethnicities have these variations in osteoporosis and fracture rates, but regardless of your ethnicity, your doctor and you need to figure out the best prevention efforts for you personally, especially if you have multiple other risk factors.

Medications That Affect Bone Density

Some medications can affect your body's ability to produce new bone or to reach its peak bone mass. Your physician can assess whether the benefit of taking these medications outweighs the risk that they may increase your chances of osteoporosis. The following sections discuss some medications that can negatively impact your bone density.

Steroids

Steroids are very strong anti-inflammatory medications that can treat conditions such as asthma, arthritis, certain auto-immune illnesses, lung disease, and psoriasis. These medications decrease the body's ability to absorb calcium. If you need to be on a steroid for longer than a few months, and at doses considered moderate to high by your prescribing healthcare provider, you have an increased risk of developing osteoporosis. Your doctor may want to prescribe a drug that helps to prevent osteoporosis at the same time that you're taking long-term steroids.

Hormone-blocking drugs

Some medications used to treat conditions such as endometriosis or breast cancer, called *hormone-blocking drugs,* can simulate a medically induced menopause. Menopause, whether medically induced or naturally occurring, increases the risk of bone thinning and osteoporosis. Depending on how long you have to take these medications, your healthcare provider may recommend additional drugs or supplements to lessen the effect of these treatments on your bones.

Diuretics

Certain medications prescribed for heart failure or high blood pressure may cause the kidneys to excrete more calcium in your urine. If this happens over a long period of time, the risk for bone loss increases. Your doctor may switch you to a different medication to treat these conditions if a urine test suggests that you're losing too much calcium in your urine.

Behaviors That Can Damage Your Bones

Genetics, age, and other factors aside, you have control over certain lifestyle changes that can help protect your bones. The following sections go into a few behaviors that definitely have a negative impact on your bone health, so if these habits are your habits consider working to change with them.

Low activity level

Exercise puts good stress on your bones, which helps your body maintain bone density. Stress on the bones forces them to absorb calcium and promotes bone strengthening. The muscles surrounding the bones also get stronger through exercise, and an improvement in overall balance can decrease the chances of a fall. These types of exercise are especially helpful in keeping your bones strong:

» **Weightbearing exercises:** During these exercises, your feet are on the ground. Walking, hiking, running, dancing, and aerobics classes all provide great bone-building, so add them into your schedule at least four or five days a week.

» **Resistance training:** Helps strengthen your bones by stressing them. Lifting weights (which don't have to be heavy), using elastic resistance bands, and even using your own body weight as resistance (such as when you do push-ups) all help prevent bone loss and may even help to build new bone.

Smoking

Although you probably know the many good reasons to quit smoking, add to that list the effect that smoking has on your bones. Smoking impairs the remodeling of bone and speeds the process of bone loss. Long-time smokers suffer more fractures from osteoporosis and take longer to heal than non-smokers.

Vaping

A study conducted by the American Journal of Medicine in 2021 revealed that individuals who engage in vaping are more prone to experiencing fragility fractures. These are fractures that occur as a result of a fall from a height lower than standing. Such fractures are commonly linked with osteoporosis.

Alcohol use

Excessive alcohol consumption decreases bone density and weakens the mechanical properties of bone. Alcohol can interfere with the balance of calcium in the bloodstream, as well as with the production of vitamin D (which is essential for calcium absorption). Alcohol can also decrease estrogen production, which can accelerate bone loss. There is evidence that consuming even one alcoholic drink per day increases the risk for osteoporosis.

Music to Your Bones: Calcium and Vitamin D

Calcium and vitamin D are two very important elements in the bone-building and remodeling story. Getting enough calcium in your diet in particular is a major part of keeping your body's ecosystem functioning, and your body needs calcium to build bone.

Getting enough calcium and vitamin D in your diet typically does not require a lot of effort, regardless of the type of diet your follow. You probably already incorporate many foods rich in calcium already.

The following sections outline the benefits of calcium and vitamin D, particularly to your bones (though also your overall health) as you experience perimenopause and lists excellent sources of both.

Upping your calcium intake

Calcium has many functions in the human body, including helping muscles to move, allowing nerves to carry messages to various parts of your body, helping blood to clot, and building and strengthening bones.

Low levels of calcium can cause fatigue, insomnia, poor dental health, brain fog, and thinning of the bones.

TIP

You can usually easily treat calcium deficiency by adding more calcium to your diet or taking calcium supplements. Discuss these changes with your doctor so that you can be sure that you're taking the proper doses. Taking too much calcium in supplement form can lead to additional health problems, such as kidney stones.

Your body's requirements for calcium level off during the reproductive years and increase around the time of perimenopause and menopause because estrogen has an effect on the body's ability to absorb calcium. When estrogen levels start to vary during perimenopause, and when they plummet after you reach menopause, you need to take in more calcium to get more calcium into your bones. Here are the recommended calcium requirements by age.

Age	Daily Calcium Recommendation
9–18	1,300 mg
19–50	1,000 mg
51 and older	1,200 mg

If the calcium in your blood drops below a certain level, the four small glands in your neck, called the *parathyroid glands* (because they are next to your thyroid gland) attempt to regulate that calcium–blood level. They send out signals to

>> The bone-destruction cells (*osteoclasts*), telling those cells to suck calcium out of the bones, which makes the bones become thinner.

>> The kidneys (where calcium is typically eliminated by sending it out of the body in urine), telling the kidneys to conserve calcium by not putting so much into urine.

When your body decides that you don't have enough calcium in your bloodstream to assist in the functions of the muscles, nerves, and heart, it goes on a mission to recoup calcium wherever it can. Your bones become one of the first victims, and you may suffer bone loss as a consequence.

How do you know how much calcium is in your foods? Most people know that dairy products have calcium, but there are many other foods that also contain calcium. It really is as simple as a math equation to figure out whether you're getting enough calcium in your diet.

TIP

Table 15-1 lists the calcium content of various foods. Look at your daily intake of these foods (or foods like them) and try to get as much as you can from dietary intake. If you are under 50 and need a total of 1,000 mg per day, supplement the rest. If you are 51 or older, you need 1,200 mg per day, and again, supplement up to that number after you add the amount that you are getting in your diet.

TABLE 15-1

Sources of Calcium in Food

Food	Standard Portion	Calcium (mg)
Dairy and Fortified Alternatives		
Almond milk	1 cup	442
Cheese	1.5 oz	115–485
Kefir	1 cup	317
1% milk	1 cup	305
Rice milk	1 cup	283
Soy milk	1 cup	301
Yogurt, plain	8 oz	488
Yogurt, Greek	8 oz	261
Vegetables, Cooked		
Bok choy	1 cup	185
Collard greens	1 cup	268
Dandelion greens	1 cup	147
Kale	1 cup	177
Mustard greens	1 cup	165
Nopales	1 cup	244
Spinach	1 cup	245
Turnip greens	1 cup	197

(continued)

TABLE 15-1 *(continued)*

Food	Standard Portion	Calcium (mg)
Proteins		
Salmon, canned	3 oz	181
Sardines, canned	3 oz	325
Tahini	1 Tbl	154
Tofu with calcium sulfate	1/2 cup	434
Fruit juices		
Grapefruit juice, fortified	1 cup	350
Orange juice, fortified	1 cup	349

With a little help from Vitamin D

Vitamin D, also called *calciferol*, doesn't occur naturally in many foods. The human body produces vitamin D when ultraviolet light rays from the sun strike the skin and trigger its synthesis. Vitamin D helps the body absorb and retain calcium and phosphorus, two minerals that are critical for building new bone. When your body doesn't have enough vitamin D (known as *vitamin D deficiency*), you can have issues with your bones and muscles. You probably need to get enough vitamin D by taking supplements because you can get such a limited amount from food (and because healthcare providers don't really recommend that people sit out in the sun).

Lack of vitamin D can cause or contribute to

>> Fatigue

>> Bone pain

>> Muscle weakness

>> Mood changes, such as depression

>> Kidney disease

>> Obesity

FINDING OUT WHERE YOUR BONES STAND

The test to diagnose thinning bones, to determine whether you may already have osteopenia or even osteoporosis, is called a *DEXA bone density test.* This test uses a targeted X-ray to evaluate bone density at several key areas in the body. It checks out the bone density of the spine, the hips, and sometimes the wrists, because these areas are the most likely to fracture. In the U.S., doctors recommend that you have this test done for the first time at age 60, unless you have some of the risk factors I talk about in the section "Medications That Affect Bone Density," in this chapter.

Prior to having a DEXA test to diagnose bone loss, focus on preventing osteoporosis by evaluating and managing your individual risk factors. Digging deeply into your family history, as well as looking at your eating habits, lifestyle choices, and supplement intake, can provide you with a game plan to prevent and battle bone loss. If you actively start managing your risks and put a plan in place to maintain your bone density while you're still in perimenopause, your menopausal years will be filled with dancing and standing tall instead of recovering from fractures that could have been prevented.

You can purchase vitamin D3 (*cholecalciferol*) over the counter, and your body can easily absorb it through your GI system. A healthcare provider can tell you exactly how much vitamin D3 you need to supplement, depending on your age and medical conditions, but the usual supplements vary from 400 to 1,200 international units (IUs) a day.

IN THIS CHAPTER

» **Keeping up-to-date with vaccinations**

» **Identifying diseases**

» **Monitoring your blood pressure and cholesterol levels**

» **Screenings for cancers**

» **Considering other useful tests and screenings**

Chapter **16**

Monitoring Your Health with Tests and Screenings

While women progress into their 40s and 50s, health needs and priorities shift, as do the screening tests that your healthcare provider may order. A primary care doctor can order or do some of these tests, and your gynecologist may do others. Go into a doctor's appointment with a list of screening tests that you want to do and discuss with your doctor which ones they recommend and why.

No medical societies consider blood tests to check hormone levels screening tests, and they don't recommend these tests for perimenopausal women. In perimenopause, hormone levels fluctuate wildly, so a blood sample taken at one point in time can't provide useful information about medically managing perimenopausal symptoms.

This chapter covers the screening tests and medical procedures that women in their early 40s to late 50s should have done to ensure optimal wellbeing and proactive healthcare management, and what you can figure out from the results.

Considering Vaccinations and Immunity

If you haven't received a vaccination against the diseases for which safe and effective vaccines are available, get up to date at your doctor's office, or a pharmacy or clinic:

>> **Measles, mumps, and rubella (also called German measles):** A blood test can tell if you have immunity to these diseases. If you don't, get the vaccine!

>> **Tetanus, diphtheria, and pertussis:** Doctors recommend a booster shot for these illnesses every 10 years.

>> **Flu:** New versions of these vaccines come out yearly to protect against the latest strains of influenza.

>> **Shingles:** If you're over 50, consider being vaccinated against shingles, which is a viral infection that can cause a painful rash on the body.

REMEMBER

No one likes getting vaccines, but getting these diseases is far worse.

Looking for Common Conditions

Women in perimenopause can be susceptible for certain conditions, including the following.

Type 2 diabetes

All adults who are *overweight* (defined as having a BMI between 25 and 29) or suffer from *obesity* (those who have a BMI of 30 or higher), as well as all adults over the age of 45, should get checked for diabetes during their yearly physical examination.

Several different tests can screen for this disease, and early diagnosis leads to earlier treatment.

Type 2 diabetes, the most common form of diabetes and most often diagnosed in people over 40 years of age, is a condition where the body can't properly utilize insulin, leading to high sugar levels in the bloodstream. If untreated, Type 2 diabetes can lead to heart disease, kidney damage, poor circulation, vision problems, and stroke.

Depression

Your healthcare provider should periodically screen you for mental health issues, especially depression, at minimum during your yearly medical examination. You might have to fill out a short screening form (such as the Patient Health Questionnaire-9, or PHQ-9), and the answers that you provide to several specific questions may identify whether you're at risk of or currently suffering from clinical depression.

Only after you have an accurate diagnosis can you get effective treatment and follow-up care.

Checking Your Organ Function

Around the age of perimenopause, it's a good idea to check to see how your organs are fuctiontioning. Here are some recommended tests to consider.

Blood pressure

Your doctor should check your blood pressure at every appointment — and at minimum, annually. According to current blood pressure guidelines, *high blood pressure* is defined as any persistent blood pressure reading where the top number (called the *systolic pressure*) is over 120 or the bottom number (the *diastolic pressure*) is over 80.

If you have consistently high blood pressure, there are guidelines for you to follow to bring it down.

High blood pressure can lead to heart attacks, kidney disease, and damage to blood vessels all over the body, especially in your head and your brain.

Lipid panel

Anyone at risk for coronary artery disease should be screened for high cholesterol levels because elevated cholesterol levels can cause narrowing of the blood vessels, stroke, heart attack, pain in the legs while walking, and chest pain.

Here are some things that put you at risk for coronary artery disease:

>> Smoking

>> High blood pressure (discussed in the preceding section)

>> Diabetes (see the section "Type 2 diabetes," earlier in this chapter)

>> Being *overweight* (having a BMI between 25 and 29) or *obese* (having a BMI of 30 or over)

>> A family history of stroke, heart attack, or other cardiac diseases

>> Lack of physical activity

>> High stress

Here are the ideal cholesterol numbers, according to the Cleveland Clinic:

>> **Total cholesterol:** Aim for under 200 milligrams per deciliter (mg/dL).

>> **HDL:** This good cholesterol should be above 60 mg/dL.

>> **LDL:** You want the bad cholesterol below 100 mg/dL.

>> **Triglycerides:** Keep these fats in the bloodstream under 150 mg/dL.

If you can't get your cholesterol levels into normal ranges by using diet, exercise, and lifestyle changes, your doctor may recommend a medication to help.

Watching Out for Cancers

The following section discusses certain cancers that doctors recommend women test for around the age of perimenopause.

Colorectal cancer

Colorectal cancer rates for people under 50 are on the rise. The American Cancer Society recommends that people who have average risk (no family history of nor symptoms of colon cancer) begin screening for colorectal cancer at age 45. Symptoms of colon cancer include

>> Blood in the stool

>> Change in bowel habits

>> Unintentional weight loss

If you have any of these symptoms, get checked when the symptoms arise, regardless of your age.

REMEMBER

Your healthcare provider has several options for colorectal screening tests, and each test can provide different results and information about your colon health:

>> **FIT test:** *FIT* stands for *fecal immunochemical testing.* This at-home test checks for blood in the stool. It is about 80 percent accurate at detecting colon cancers.

>> **Cologuard test:** This at-home DNA test looks for biomarkers in your stool sample; doctors recommend it for people over 45 who are at average risk for colon cancer. One study showed it detected over 90 percent of colon cancers in people who completed the test.

>> **Colonoscopy:** This test is done in a hospital or surgical center, and includes sedation or general anesthesia. It involves a medical provider using a flexible camera to visualize the inside of the rectum and intestines. You need to go through a day of colon clean-out to prepare for the test, and you need several hours to recover from the medications used during the test. The results of this test are about 98 percent accurate in detecting colon cancers.

TIP

When you have a colonoscopy to screen for cancer, the doctor performing the exam can usually remove any polyps or growths that they see. Doctors recommend a colonoscopy every ten years for everyone over 45 years old, although studies show that only about 35 percent of people who should have the screening actually do.

REMEMBER

The tests in the preceding list aren't all equal in diagnosing colon cancer. A colonoscopy is the recommended test, and if a colonoscopy is negative, you can do other tests in the ten years between colonoscopies.

Breast cancer

A *mammogram*, an X-ray of the breasts, is the most common screening test for breast cancer, starting at age 40 for women at average risk. A mammogram can detect many small early breast cancers.

According to the National Cancer Institute, women should have the option to have a mammogram every year until age 55; and then some women should screen less often if they don't want a yearly exam (and if their doctor agrees). A discussion with your physician regarding your risks and screening results can help you figure out how often to have a mammogram, and whether other diagnostic tests (such as ultrasounds and MRIs) can benefit your screening regimen.

REMEMBER

It used to be the medical community recommended that women do a self-breast exam every month to check for lumps and bumps. Now, most medical organizations don't recommend routine self-breast exams as a part of breast cancer screening. But doctors do believe that you should be familiar with your breasts so that you can report any changes promptly.

Cervical cancer

About 13,000 new cases of cervical cancer are diagnosed in the United States every year. The *cervix* is the lower, narrow end of the uterus that connects the uterus to the vagina.

The main risk factor for cervical cancer is the presence of human papilloma virus (HPV). This virus is sexually transmitted, and in addition to cervical cancer, it can cause vaginal, vulvar, penile, and throat cancer. Cervical cancer is the only type of cancer caused by HPV that doctors can detected in its early stages by using a screening test.

HPV testing is usually paired with a *Pap smear,* a test that looks for cervical cancer, and the intervals between testing depend on your personal risk factors. All women should have Pap smears between the ages of 21 and 65, unless they no longer have their cervix. (When a woman has a hysterectomy, the surgeon often also removes the cervix — but not always.)

How often you need a pap smear depends on many factors, such as if you've ever had an Pap smear result, if you have a compromised immune system, and the number of sexual partners you've had in your lifetime.

Additional Screening Tests

Your primary care physician or other healthcare provider may suggest ordering these tests for you:

» **Full-body skin check:** About 9,000 new cases of skin cancer are diagnosed in the U.S. every day. Regularly having someone check the skin all over your body, especially in places that you can't easily see, means that you can identify any changes early on.

» **Thyroid screen:** One of the hallmarks of perimenopause is irregular periods. Because hormone levels vary widely, bleeding patterns can seem to get out of control. The thyroid gland plays a major role in the body's metabolism. When the thyroid isn't working properly, it may affect the release of hormones, causing irregular bleeding. A blood test can reveal thyroid hormone levels, so talk with your medical provider and determine whether your thyroid is functioning normally.

» **Complete blood count (CBC):** Heavy bleeding can also cause *anemia* (a low amount of *hemoglobin,* or iron-rich red blood cells, in your blood); a *CBC* is a

Chapter **17**

Ten Perimenopause Myths Exposed

When women talk to other women about their mid-life experiences, one question gets repeated often: "Why didn't anyone ever tell me about this?"

The truth is, until recently, you might struggle to find reliable information and education about what exactly happens while you go through the transition from your reproductive years to your menopausal years. However, you can find many misconceptions out there; friends, relatives, and online sources freely offer incorrect information (either because they want to help or because they want to sell you something).

This lack of solid information may make you feel even less prepared to face the many life changes that go along with perimenopause. In this chapter, I evaluate and dispel some of the myths of perimenopause.

You Can't Use Hormones When in Perimenopause

The definition of *menopause* is 12 months without a menstrual period; menopause usually happens around the age of 51, and it typically comes with symptoms such as hot flashes, insomnia, vaginal dryness, low energy, and low libido.

Many women begin to experience these symptoms well before they have reached the 12-month-no-period time frame. One of the unfortunate realities of perimenopause is that you may experience many of the annoying and irritating symptoms of your younger years (heavy and irregular bleeding, emotional mood swings) at the very same time (sometimes in the very same day) that you experience symptoms of menopause.

A medical practitioner experienced in treating menopausal and perimenopausal women listens to your symptoms — all of your symptoms — and comes up with a plan that can relieve them. This plan may or may not include hormones or hormonal contraception. Your doctor and you need to come up with a plan specific and individualized to your needs and your medical history. Sometimes, women go through the perimenopausal transition for years. If medical professionals had to just wait for the periods to end for 12 months in order to treat, many women with exasperating midlife symptoms would have to live with their suffering untreated for years.

TIP

If your periods stop completely much earlier than age 51, talk to your doctor. They need to evaluate *premature menopause* (menopause that occurs prior to age 42) to figure out whether they can identify a cause as to why your ovaries stopped working earlier than usual. Premature menopause may put you at risk for other medical problems, such as heart disease and osteoporosis.

Expect a Lower Sex Drive (and Less Satisfaction)

Say whaaaaaat? Although you may start to feel a little less interested in sex, need more sleep, or require a little more stimulation at this age, don't think that you have to kiss your sex life goodbye. Women at midlife can be sexy and sexual; they can have satisfying sexual activity by themselves or with a partner (or two) and can explore new techniques, no matter their age. (See Chapter 7 for the rundown of your sex life at midlife.)

Irregular Vaginal Bleeding Is a Danger Sign

In your perimenopausal years, irregular vaginal bleeding is usually the norm, not a sign of something dangerous. The fluctuating hormone levels during perimenopause, along with the lack of regular ovulations, conspire to create a signaling pathway between the brain, the ovaries, and the uterus that results in irregular bleeding. Many women don't know exactly when or if their period will make an appearance. Keeping track of exactly what type of period pattern you experience, over the course of a specific period of time, gives you important information to present to your doctor.

Although some bleeding patterns might raise red flags, in general, disruptions and changes in period bleeding patterns relate to the natural hormonal swings that occur in the midlife transition. Ultimately, the periods stop, and after you go through 12 consecutive months without menstrual bleeding, you're typically done with that mess forever. (See Chapter 6 for the details on perimenopause menstrual bleeding.)

You Can't Have Menopausal Symptoms in Perimenopause

The hallmark of perimenopause is to have many different and varied symptoms that seem to have no pattern other than that they consistently cause you discomfort. The span of time where you may be skipping periods, getting more frequent periods, or having menstrual bleeding patterns that seem unusual to you may last for years. Just because you still experience periods with any kind of regularity (or irregularity) doesn't mean that the symptoms of hot flashes, night sweats, insomnia, low energy, mood swings, low libido, and vaginal dryness (among others) are not very real!

Symptoms can also come and go; you may experience several months of night sweats and think, "It may be time to go see my doctor." But those symptoms may resolve for several months before they return. The only certainty about perimenopause is the uncertainty of the symptoms. You don't need a clear idea of what's going on to justify a visit to your doctor to get relief — they're there to help you figure that out.

Everyone Leaks Urine While They Age

First of all, it's *not* a given that your bladder won't work as efficiently while you age. Bladder health depends on so many things: general health, nutrition, weight, diet, number and type of pregnancies and deliveries, bathroom habits, alcohol consumption, and fluid intake, to name just a few.

As discussed in Chapter 8, which gets into all the details of the midlife bladder, you may encounter several different bladder problems while you age, but you have many things that you can do to relieve them. Adult diaper commercials may tell you not to worry because you can always wear one and go about your business, but please don't believe that's your only solution! Have an evaluation with your medical provider and explore ways to treat bladder dysfunction, regardless of what urinary issue is stressing you out — leakage, urgency, nighttime waking, or something else.

If You Maintain a Healthy Diet and Exercise, You Won't Gain Weight

You may feel puzzled because you're doing all the same things that you've been doing to stay at a healthy weight — eating salads, staying away from candy, exercising regularly, and not visiting fast food restaurants — but your weight continues to creep up. Studies show that women do gain about 2 to 5 pounds during the perimenopausal transition.

This weight gain can occur for a couple of reasons:

>> **Increased appetite:** You may experience an increase in appetite thanks to the hormonal changes that occur in midlife.

>> **Decreased estrogen levels:** Low estrogen levels may contribute to weight gain, especially around the middle.

In short, you may need to make changes to both your diet and exercise habits during perimenopause to prevent weight gain and a loss of muscle mass.

5

The Part of Tens

blood test that measures the number and type of cells in your blood, including red blood cells that carry iron.

You have to have a very low iron level in your blood before you start to feel symptoms of anemia (such as dizziness or shortness of breath). Checking your blood count regularly to make sure that you don't have anemia can let you know if you have a problem before you suffer major symptoms. If your CBC reveals that you have anemia or iron deficiency, you can treat it with dietary changes or iron replacement.

REMEMBER

A low blood count may also prompt your healthcare provider to conduct an investigation into reasons for anemia other than menstrual bleeding.

>> **Metabolic panel:** You may need to check that your kidneys and liver are functioning normally. A metabolism panel blood test can reveal kidney disease and electrolyte abnormalities. It can also screen for high blood sugar, a component of diabetes (see the section "Type 2 diabetes," earlier in this chapter).

>> **Screening for sexually transmitted infections (STIs):** If you potentially have an infection that you can transmit sexually, get yourself screened. Many STIs have no symptoms but do have major consequences. If you have a new sexual partner, have multiple partners, or have sex with someone who has additional partners (especially if any of this sex is unprotected), ask your doctor to test for

- Chlamydia

- Gonorrhea

- Hepatitis B and C

- HIV

- Syphilis

You Just Have to Wait It Out

If your symptoms are mild and require minimal changes in your daily activities to relieve them (open the windows if you have hot flashes, use different sheets on your bed for night sweats), then you may breeze through your perimenopausal transition without much disruption. Most symptoms, especially mild ones, do eventually resolve.

However, if you have severe, life-altering perimenopausal symptoms, don't think that you just have to wait it out. This book arms you with information that you can present to your doctor, and together, you can create a plan to deal with your symptoms for however long you experience them.

Also, some symptoms, such vaginal dryness, will never improve without continued attention. As discussed in Chapter 7, the vagina has many receptors for estrogen, and without supplemental estrogen or some type of vaginal moisturizer, thinning and dryness of vaginal tissue will continue to worsen. Don't just wait this one out.

You Don't Need to See a Doctor Unless You Have a Big Problem

For some unknown reason, many women have this idea that they should "tough it out" when it comes to perimenopausal symptoms. They may or may not consult their friends or the Internet, but they generally wait until their quality of life is really suffering to seek true medical help. They buy over-the-counter remedies for their hot flashes. They download apps to advise them on how to fix their insomnia or their anxiety. They may have multiple irritating symptoms that actually have simple solutions, but they don't feel the need (or the right) to ask for help.

Don't wait! Go to your doctor and raise your concerns. Your healthcare provider can evaluate your problems and help you find solutions to them before those problems become overwhelming.

You Need Blood Tests to Check Your Hormones

One of the myths that continually appears in online discussion groups is the recommendation to check your hormone levels in order to effectively treat your symptoms. The truth is, medical providers almost always decide on treatments for perimenopausal and menopausal symptoms by listening to your symptoms and taking a good history. You don't get any real benefit from determining your hormone-level numbers and then using some form of treatment to attempt to change these numbers.

REMEMBER

You can find some exceptions to this rule: If your symptoms seem unusual for your age, if you're not responding to treatment (meaning you aren't experiencing relief from your symptoms), or if your doctor is treating you with testosterone, they may want to do a few blood tests to evaluate your hormone levels.

But no medical society recommends treating symptoms by drawing blood and basing treatment plans solely on the results of these hormonal blood tests. In perimenopause, these hormone levels vary by the week — or even by the day. So the numbers you get from one blood test can't provide useful information to help you and your doctor create an effective hormone treatment plan.

Perimenopause Doesn't Happen Until You're Too Old to Have a Baby

Most women experience perimenopause between the ages of 43 and 52, at a time during which they still may be ovulating. Although you probably don't have to worry about becoming pregnant in the perimenopausal period, a pregnancy can still happen unless you go through 12 consecutive months without a period. Remember — a missed period can be a sign of pregnancy until proven otherwise. If you're sexually active in perimenopause and don't want a pregnancy, use an effective method of birth control, always.

Chapter **18**

Ten Things to Ignore During Perimenopause

When women feel unprepared and uninformed, they seek out helpful information. The sources of this information for perimenopausal women are often discussions with friends and family members who have already experienced perimenopause (and may already be in menopause) or reading printed or online resources. The available information may give you conflicting and confusing advice.

Every woman may experience different symptoms during this phase of life. No one has a one-size-fits-all remedy or approach to perimenopause that works for everyone. Even well-meaning people can end up giving advice or making comments that, at best, don't offer you much help or, at worst, are dismissive and hurtful.

Also, marketers understand that women eagerly want relief from their perimenopausal symptoms, and they can target you with products and therapies that may not be helpful — and that actually may be harmful.

Perimenopause and misinformation often go hand in hand, so this chapter offers some things that you can usually ignore while you go through your midlife changes and challenges.

Women Who Say, "That Didn't Happen to Me!"

Your experiences while you go through perimenopause are unique and your own. Your perimenopause experience or experiences won't be exactly like anyone else's, even if that person is biologically closely connected to you, such as your mom or your twin sister.

REMEMBER

Although many women going through perimenopause share some symptoms, the way in which you experience these symptoms and the degree to which they affect your life depends on the uniqueness of you.

Even though you can listen to your family history or to friends' experiences, don't expect your experiences to be the same — and please don't think something's amiss if you have quite different symptoms or reactions. Discuss any concerns you have with your healthcare provider, and the two of you can figure out your perimenopausal normal.

Friends and Family Who Know What You Need to Do

You may hear it all the time: "I had hot flashes, and I started on hormone replacement therapy." Or "I couldn't sleep, so I tried CBD gummies."

These people mean well and want to share their journey with you because they finally found something that worked for them. But they don't know your medical history, your allergies, or your (sometimes complex) medication list. What worked for them may work for you — or it may be totally unsafe for you because of these missing pieces of information. Take the advice with a smile and a grain of salt and take the list of suggestions to your medical provider so that they can help you decide what suggestion or combination of suggestions you can safely include in your plan.

Advertisers Who Promise Miraculous Weight Loss

I'm sure you've heard the advice, "If it sounds too good to be true, it probably is." You can find thousands of weight loss supplements, pills, and detoxes available on the market. Even if your doctor puts you on one of the newer weight loss medications that you hear mentioned in the news all the time, losing weight and maintaining a healthy weight take some work and effort for most women while they go through perimenopause.

No one has a miracle drug, shot, or supplement that can safely and quickly make you thinner. Please don't waste your money on these bogus fixes. And block any social media advertisements that pop up so that they can't waste your time and attention.

Online Forums That Tell You to Ignore Your Doctor's Advice (and Follow Theirs)

Countless websites, blogs, and celebrity advice columns tell you that you can have an easy and symptom-free perimenopause if you just follow their recommendations. If you dig deeper, you often find that these advice-givers aren't doctors or nurse practitioners; they're often not medical professionals at all, and certainly not specialists in the field of women's health or menopausal medicine.

Celebrities and other influencers may have stories to tell but have no stake in your health. You should see a big red flag if they give advice about your symptoms and then recommend some product — that they just happen to sell — to relieve those symptoms.

REMEMBER

A medical professional who knows you and who can evaluate you as an individual is your best bet for relieving your perimenopausal symptoms and making that transition to menopause safely.

Ads That Make You Feel Bad about Your Age or Body

Do commercials have to assume that you're unhappy with some aspect of your body to sell you a product? If the feeling that you get from an ad is that you can't be sexy or sexual because of your age or you can't be attractive because of your weight or size, don't buy those products. You can find all kinds of harmful messaging about not being thin enough or tall enough, or not having a desirable skin tone or body shape. Don't encourage this type of advertising by patronizing these companies. You may have to do a little investigating but look for companies that use realistic models and don't have marketing campaigns that leave you feeling less confident; send a message that you want to spend your money on a company with a positive message.

Anyone Who Expects You to Sacrifice Yourself for Them

In perimenopause, you fall into the sandwich generation. Aging parents often require more time and care, while children may not have moved out on their own yet. Sometimes, after college, children move back in, convinced that their parents are oh-so-happy to have them back.

In truth, empty nesters may look forward to this time as one of self-care and alone time (with or without a partner). Bearing responsibility for aging parents and needy children can lead to a lot of stress, which can lead to poor health.

TIP

Perfect your self-care skills, along with your ability to say no to some of the burdens that seem so automatically assigned to you. Enlist outside help, whether you get that help from other family members or from professionals, and remember that if you don't take care of yourself, you can't take care of anyone else. Believe it, and act accordingly.

Healthcare Professionals Who Don't Know Perimenopause

A whole specialty in women's health focuses on women in midlife and beyond. Healthcare providers (doctors, nurse practitioners, and physician's assistants, among others) who study the subject and take an exam about the specifics of menopause and perimenopause management can earn Nationally Certified Menopause Practitioner (NCMP) certification.

Many gynecologists, whether they take this exam or not, are skilled in the management of midlife issues. And family practitioners and internists may also take a special interest in treating women at these life stages. You may need to enlist a combination of practitioners to take care of several different problems in perimenopause.

WARNING

If your doctor doesn't act on your perimenopause concerns and doesn't offer you solutions for your perimenopausal symptoms, find another healthcare provider. You may have to do a little investigating and research to find the help you deserve but knowing that the right provider can help you find solutions will make the effort worth it.

Anyone Who Thinks You Have to Fit a Mold

Perimenopause is exactly the time to have less concern about living according to the expectations of others. Who cares if someone thinks you can no longer be fun, sexy, energetic, or silly? You don't have time in your day or energy to respond to anyone who wants to hold you to an "age-appropriate" standard of behavior. You can use this time to reinvent yourself, reassessing what you find important in your life and keeping a distance from anyone who makes you feel miserable or inferior.

Anyone Who Says Depression or Anxiety Are Normal in Perimenopause

Some emotional and mental health issues may accompany perimenopause, or those issues might become more pronounced during perimenopause (which you can read about in Chapter 10, where I talk about your mental health during perimenopause). But don't believe that continuing symptoms of anxiety and depression come as just a part of the change:

>> **Anxiety:** If you feel anxious about everyday activities, or if your anxiety causes poor sleep, investigate these feelings further with the help of a medical professional.

>> **Depression:** If you find yourself experiencing sad feelings, which may be accompanied by appetite changes, sleeping too much, and not getting pleasure from activities that you previously enjoyed, discuss these feelings with a healthcare provider to determine whether you're suffering from depression.

REMEMBER

Never discount or ignore mental and emotional health issues as normal at any stage of life; you may have more difficulty separating perimenopausal symptoms from psychological disorders, but a skilled professional can help you do so.

Any Thoughts That Keep You from Seeking Professional Help

For some reason, women usually suffer with symptoms for weeks or months before deciding to seek help because they think they need to "tough it out." This inaction can happen for several reasons:

>> Maybe you feel that the symptoms are only temporary.

>> You might reason that, compared to other women, your symptoms aren't that bad.

>> You may just not know where to turn.

REMEMBER

You're worth the effort of seeking help. You deserve to feel better. If you need help to think of the rest of your life as an opportunity and not a sentence, get it. You can treat the symptoms of perimenopause with help from your healthcare provider. You just need to turn off the chatter, listen to yourself (and this book!), and seek the care that you deserve.

Chapter **19**

Ten Things You *Really* Need During Perimenopause

This chapter lists for you the bare minimum that you must have in your toolbox to help you make it through your perimenopausal transition healthy, happy, and filled with optimism.

Reliable, Accurate Information

This book and others, as well as websites and videos, have accurate and interesting information that you can use to help navigate the midlife years. You need to be able to tell the good information from the bad and differentiate the informative practitioners from the salespeople. (See Appendix B for my recommendations for good resources.)

Outlets for Pleasure and Relaxation

Whether you go for a hobby, a sport, a book, a garden, an exercise class, a group of friends, volunteer work, or anything else, find something to look forward to every day or every week that you enjoy participating in. (If you can't find pleasure in anything, please see Chapter 10, which discusses how to care for your mental health during perimenopause.)

A Regular Good Night's Sleep

I don't have much more to say on getting a good night's sleep; it's something that you absolutely need to stay healthy, regardless of what phase of life you're in. If you can't get good sleep, most of the time, anything else that you do to try to keep yourself happy and healthy doesn't matter. Poor sleep creates poor health, so seek out whichever method or combination of methods can help you get a good night's rest.

A Good Listener

You need someone to talk to during these very stressful years. Whether you can rely on conversations with a friend, family member, therapist, counselor, or neighbor, make sure that you have someone who can offer support and understanding — or just a listening ear.

A Trustworthy Healthcare Provider

Ideally, prior to your perimenopausal years, you find a gynecologist, primary care doctor, nurse practitioner, or other healthcare provider who knows about midlife changes and can help you along the journey when the time comes.

The same person who treated your coughs and colds when you were younger, or even the person who delivered your babies, probably can't fill that midlife need (although they might).

When you begin going through perimenopause (or suspect that you are), find a practitioner who knows the intricacies and specifics of midlife changes. And if that need means that you have to find someone new, that's okay.

A Healthy Eating Plan

Create an eating plan that supports good physical and mental health. Don't even call it a diet. The word *diet* makes you think of restrictions and all the foods that you can't have.

Think of this eating plan as a way to really find out how to eat and drink the things that can help keep you healthy and help you live longer for the rest of your life. It's never too late to change your habits — and making healthy food changes a little at a time can slowly improve the quality of your life.

A Plan to Maintain Strong Bones

If you don't want to be wrapped in a cast, lose height, or end up with a hump on your back, take care of your bones before any of that happens. A fractured hip can change your ability to be independent, and it can also change the quality and the length of your life.

Lifestyle, exercise, nutrition, supplements, and sometimes medication can combine to maintain bone strength and decrease your risk for life-changing fractures.

A List (and a Schedule) of Recommended Health Screenings

You absolutely need to know what health challenges you may be facing during perimenopause; the only way to keep tabs on your health involves working with your doctor to set up recommended tests and screenings. You don't have a ton of tests to set up, so get them done.

Checking out the current state of your health gives you (and your doctor) an idea of where you are and where you're headed. Together, you can treat any medical condition, improve your health, and stay informed for your future. (See Chapter 15 for more information on staying informed about your health with tests and screenings.)

A Sunproof Skincare Routine

By the time you're in perimenopause, you're at increased risk for skin cancer because of the number of years that you probably allowed your skin to be exposed to the sun without adequate protection. (If you've been a diehard SPF user from your early years, kudos!) Avoid ultraviolet (UV) radiation from the sun as much as possible. And when you are out in the sun, always wear sunscreen of at least SPF 50 on all exposed areas. Drink plenty of water and apply a daily moisturizer to your skin.

A (Realistic) Plan to Keep Your Body Moving

If you don't have time for a workout, hate sweat, and feel like exercise requires just too much effort, you need to change your perspective. If you haven't yet, make some type of exercise as routine as brushing your teeth. Whether you walk, run, swim, stair-climb, do elliptical training, cycle, practice yoga, or do Pilates, everyone can find something that they can do four to five days a week, for 20 to 30 minutes at a time. In our multitasking society, you can often do two things at the same time: Listen to a podcast or talk to a friend while you take a walk; watch a show while you use a treadmill. But you must move, or one day you'll find that you can't.

Chapter **20**

Ten Perimenopause Stories from My Practice

find in my work that women gain comfort from hearing stories about other women who are going through similar health issues. Whether the woman is going through pregnancy, menstruation, perimenopause, or some other stage in life, information from the experiences of other women can give you perspective. These stories can also provide information on available treatment plans for your ongoing symptoms.

In my years of practice, I've met with and treated many women experiencing the hormonal chaos of perimenopause, and I can assert absolutely that no two cases are exactly alike — and therefore no one-size-fits-all solution or cure exists. I often think women would feel more confident about sharing their symptoms if they understood how common those symptoms are in perimenopause and how the right personalized plan can help provide relief.

This chapter offers a look at some of the very real perimenopausal women I have encountered. But even if a case sounds very much like what you're going through, always see your doctor to help determine the best treatment plan for you. These cases do, however, illustrate how thinking outside of the standard hormone-therapy box can lead to a more appropriate and personalized treatment plan, and why it's always worth seeking a second opinion if you feel that your own doctor suggests treatments that aren't working for you.

When Polyps Are the Problem

A 46-year-old patient came to see me for a new patient appointment. She told me that for the past six months, she had been getting her period every two weeks, and it was heavy and crampy. She had had tubal ligation (a procedure in which the fallopian tubes are permanently blocked or disconnected so that eggs can't travel from the ovaries into the tubes, thus preventing pregnancy), so she didn't need contraception to prevent pregnancy. She told me that a doctor had removed some polyps from her uterus several years ago, and her periods had been very regular until six months ago. I took a full history and did a physical exam, ordered some labs (which were all normal), and scheduled a hysteroscopy, a procedure where I look with a small camera inside the uterus.

Sure enough, I found some polyps in the uterine cavity, which I removed. Her periods went back to monthly, and she was happy to not need to use hormones or any other unnecessary medications just to correct the frequent periods. Hormones don't cause all the changes in menstrual patterns during perimenopause!

Relieving Hot Flashes and Depressive Symptoms

A 49-year-old woman presented to my office, reporting that her periods came every two to four months, and in between, she had hot flashes and poor sleep. She also stated that she felt symptoms of depression regularly. After a thorough discussion of her medical history, life circumstances, and the medications she was taking, we figured out that she wasn't really bothered by the irregular periods, but the hot flashes and depression were her main stressors.

We came up with a plan to use venlafaxine (a serotonin boosting anti-depressant, brand name Effexor), which can help relieve hot flashes as well as depressive symptoms. (Of course, we also discussed diet, exercise, and the benefits of a good therapist.)

This patient still would need some kind of birth control if she was sexually active because even every-few-month periods can mean every-few-month ovulations (and potential pregnancies)!

When Supplements Wreak Havoc

A 54-year-old patient had been coming to me regularly since the age of 50. At her first visit, she relayed that her last period occurred over two years ago, and she had recently seen her primary care physician for treatment of her hot flashes, poor sleep, irritability, and vaginal dryness.

Her doctor started her on escitalopram (brand name Lexapro), an antidepressant medication. (Her complaints at the time didn't include depression, and nothing in her history or physical exam suggested she couldn't start hormone therapy, but a doctor not suggesting such an option isn't an unusual scenario.)

She told me that the antidepressant made her feel like a zombie, so she discontinued it. After an exam and a discussion about possible treatments for her menopausal symptoms, she started on an estrogen patch, along with oral progesterone. This combination took care of her symptoms and caused no side effects for four years.

But after those four years, the woman came to see me reporting that she had suddenly started bleeding, similar to when she had a period. She hadn't missed any doses of her hormones but did recently start taking a supplement that she found on the Internet that contained *black cohosh*, a supplement advertised as a hot flash relief. She thought the supplement might be a good addition to her menopause plan.

Although black cohosh can sometimes act like estrogen on the uterine lining, I still had to confirm why she was bleeding. I couldn't assume it was from the new supplement because I didn't want to miss anything. I biopsied her uterus, and there was no evidence of cancerous or precancerous cells that might have caused the bleeding.

I told her to discontinue the supplement. The bleeding stopped, and we had a conversation about how supplements can have interactions with hormone therapy and medications, so to always check with her treating physician before adding anything in.

Hot Flashes Don't Always Require Hormone Therapy

A 46-year-old woman who came to see me as a new patient reported that she had gone to her general practitioner with complaints of hot flashes, fatigue, weight gain, brain fog, depression, joint pain, and low back pain. She reported still having a heavy, painful menstrual period every month that was getting heavier in the last year or so.

Without doing any testing, her doctor prescribed her an estrogen pill and a progesterone cream. I advised her to stop using these prescriptions. Although she had hot flashes, the fact that she had regular menstrual periods suggested that she was still making plenty of estrogen, and no studies suggest that a progesterone cream might safely or appropriately treat her.

We did some lab work: She had a normal thyroid and was anemic from all that bleeding. I suggested she switch to a birth control pill and start an iron supplement; we added in an antidepressant medication later to treat her depressive symptoms. Her menstrual bleeding became lighter, she had her depression under control, and with some suggested changes to her diet and exercise plan, she felt she had good relief of her symptoms.

Moral of the story: Not all hot flashes require menopausal hormone therapy. Please get your advice from a specialist in perimenopause and menopause, if you can.

Estrogen Patches to the Rescue

A 52-year-old long-time patient came to see me with new complaints of hot flashes, night sweats, and trouble sleeping. She had a progesterone-releasing IUD that I had inserted three years prior for contraception, and ever since it was placed, she didn't have another period. She wondered whether she was in menopause, and if so, whether she would need to have the IUD removed to relieve her symptoms.

I saw her situation as a very easy problem to solve. Her age, combined with her complaints of hot flashes and night sweats, gave me all the history I felt I needed to know that I could easily treat her like she was in menopause.

After discussing her medical history to be sure her situation gave me no reason not to use estrogen, I prescribed an estrogen patch. For her progesterone, she kept her IUD in place — she didn't need anything else. This easy solution relieved her symptoms and will likely take her through her perimenopausal transition and into menopause.

Discontinuing Hormones in Favor of Other Solutions

A 45-year-old patient came to see me as a new patient. She was a patient at a local HMO and was seeking gynecological care there. She gave birth to her last child five years prior, at age 40. At 45, she reported low libido, fatigue, and migraines; her other doctor had started her on testosterone and estrogen to treat these symptoms.

She then started having heavy menstrual bleeding and worsening migraines, which brought her to me. I strongly advised her to go off these hormones and allow me to do a full evaluation, with a complete history, labs (checking blood count, thyroid function, iron level, and some other blood levels), and an ultrasound of her uterus and ovaries.

After a workup and discussion of our findings, we came up with a plan that included an iron supplement, a migraine medication, and oral progesterone. Five years later, she was still on the same plan (with some minor annual adjustments) and experiencing good relief from all her symptoms.

Evaluating a Patient for Perimenopause

Several years ago, a 48-year-old woman came to me as a new patient, specifically asking "to be evaluated for perimenopause." She had had a *tubal ligation* (a form or permanent birth control where a doctor blocks or disconnects the fallopian tubes so that eggs can't travel from the ovaries into the tubes) and reported having very heavy monthly periods, with PMS symptoms, fatigue, hot flashes daily, and trouble sleeping. She also complained of vaginal dryness and pain during sex. I did my usual exam and ordered some lab work.

The lab results told me that her thyroid was normal and that she was quite anemic. I first offered her choices of hormonal birth control, which might provide the non-contraceptive benefit of lessening her periods and hot flashes, but she didn't want to use hormonal birth control.

We came up with a plan of using progesterone only in the five to seven days prior to each period, as well as an iron supplement to treat her anemia, and a good vaginal moisturizer that contained hyaluronic acid as the main ingredient to help her vaginal dryness. She did well on this plan, and we can adjust it when she becomes menopausal.

Considering Testosterone

A 55-year-old patient who had been coming to see me for five years presented for her annual checkup. Ever since age 52, she had been on a menopausal hormone therapy program, including a transdermal estrogen cream that she applied once daily, as well as an oral progesterone tablet that she would take every night before bed.

With this plan, she reported no hot flashes or night sweats, no trouble sleeping, good energy, and relief from any vaginal dryness. However, she had started to notice a decrease in her libido. She reported that this was a recent, gradual change, and it troubled her. We discussed the possibility that something identifiable might be responsible for this change: But she had no change in her happy relationship, no new medications, and no big stressors at home or at work.

Because she had been using the same estrogen dose for quite a while, I suggested raising the dose. Sometimes low libido can result from a too-low estrogen dose. I also suggested considering the addition of testosterone to her menopausal hormone therapy regimen.

After we discussed the risks and benefits and reviewed the prevailing ideas about desire (see Chapter 7 for the ins and outs of your perimenopausal sex life), we decided to try transdermal compounded testosterone. After being on the testosterone for one year, we found a dose that seemed to help, and my patient happily remained on the trio of estrogen, progesterone, and testosterone for her menopausal hormone therapy (MHT) management.

Detecting Precancerous Cells

A 49-year-old new patient came to my office to be evaluated for a complaint of heavy, constant vaginal bleeding. By taking a thorough history, I found out that this patient had gone to a clinic that was advertised as a specialty menopause clinic.

She had a consultation with a practitioner, and they drew a lot of blood. They told her that she had very low estrogen and testosterone levels, and that her adrenal glands were fatigued. The clinic sold her some supposed adrenal-support supplements and placed several hormonal pellets under her skin, one containing estrogen and one containing testosterone.

She did report to me, two months later, that immediately after the pellet placement, she did have more energy and fewer hot flashes. However, less than a month after that, she started having vaginal bleeding that became heavier and more painful. She had been experiencing this heavy bleeding for weeks, and when she called the menopause clinic back, they advised her to find a gynecologist to see her.

I did a full exam, a pelvic ultrasound, and a biopsy of the lining inside the uterus (an *endometrial* biopsy). We discovered that she had a precancerous condition in the lining of the uterus called *complex atypical hyperplasia*. I referred her to a *gynecologic oncologist* (a doctor who specializes in cancers of the female reproductive system), who performed a *hysterectomy* (surgical removal of the uterus).

Luckily, the condition hadn't yet developed into cancer, and she recovered well from the surgery. I still care for this patient, using safe methods to relieve her hot flashes and other menopausal symptoms.

Treatment Options with a Family Breast Cancer History

A 49-year-old patient came to me recently for her first visit. She reported having gone to her primary care doctor with complaints of hot flashes and night sweats, as well as recent brain fog and forgetfulness. She'd had a progesterone-releasing IUD placed three years prior and had immediately stopped having periods, but the hot flashes and brain fog symptoms had just started a few months ago.

Her primary care doctor advised her that she was not a candidate to start menopausal hormone therapy because her mother had had breast cancer. After getting a thorough history, it turned out that this patient's mother had had breast cancer at age 50 but had not been tested for genetic mutations for breast cancer, such as the BRCA gene. So my patient could do the genetic test if she wanted to help us figure out her risk for breast cancer and make our decisions accordingly.

Meanwhile, I offered her alternatives to hormone therapy for her hot flashes, poor sleep, and brain fog. We started her on a prescription medication called fezolinetant to treat the hot flashes and night sweats. By getting relief from hot flashes and night sweats, and therefore better sleep, her concentration improved, and her brain fog lessened. We discussed altering her diet and increasing her exercise, and then we set up an appointment for her to return to be tested for a genetic risk for breast cancer.

REMEMBER

If this patient tested positive as a carrier of a genetic mutation that increases her risk for breast and ovarian cancer, we don't necessarily have to rule out her ability to use menopausal hormone therapy (MHT); she and I — doctor and patient — will make that decision together.

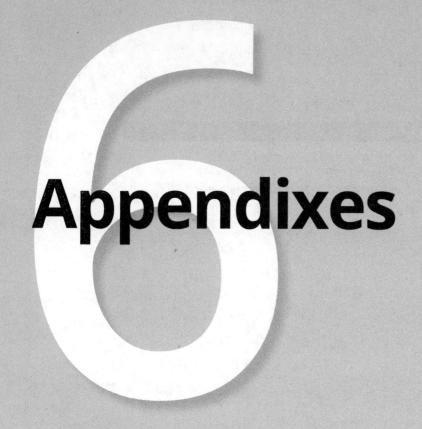

Appendixes

Learn key terms related to perimenopause.

Find out where to look for more information and support.

Appendix A

Glossary

Amenorrhea: A condition in which menstrual periods stop. Many things can cause this condition, including genetics, hormone changes, surgery, and stress. See also *menses*.

Androgens: Hormones that produce masculine effects on the body; produced in the adrenal glands of both men and women, also by the ovaries in women and in the testicles in men. Women usually produce androgens in much smaller amounts than men. See also *hormone*.

Atherosclerosis: A type of blocking or damage to the *arteries* (blood vessels that carry blood away from the heart) that causes narrowing and difficulty bringing blood to the rest of the body. It can lead to *coronary artery disease,* a disease of the blood vessels of the heart.

Atrophic vaginitis: An outdated term for *Genitourinary Syndrome of Menopause (GSM).*

Bilateral salpingo-oophorectomy: Surgical removal of both ovaries and fallopian tubes. See also, *fallopian tubes, oophorectomy, ovaries.*

Bisphosphonates: A class of drugs used for osteoporosis prevention and treatment. They slow down bone destruction and breakdown. See also *osteoporosis.*

Blood pressure: The force of blood against the walls of the arteries while the heart pumps blood through the body. Medical professionals typically measure blood pressure with two numbers: systolic, which has a normal of about 120 millimeters of mercury (mmHg, a measure of pressure) or below; and diastolic (normal 80 mmHg or below). See also *hypertension.*

Body mass index (BMI): A formula for estimating total body fat by using a weight-to-height ratio. It's based primarily on data collected from previous generations of non-Hispanic white populations, and many weight management specialists feel it is not a valid measure of overall health despite its continued use in medical practice.

BRCA1 and BRCA2: Abbreviation for BReast CAncer susceptibility genes, which are responsible for controlling cell growth and suppression of cancer cells. Inheritance of an abnormal version of one of these genes raises your risk of developing breast and ovarian cancer.

Cervix: The lower part of the uterus, which connects to the top of the vagina. See also *uterus, vagina.*

Cholesterol: A fat-like substance that comprises an important part of the body's cells. Cholesterol performs many normal functions in the body. When you have normal levels of cholesterol in your bloodstream, the body uses it in building hormones and new blood cells. Cholesterol comes from two sources: your liver, and the foods that you eat. (Your liver actually makes all the cholesterol that you need.)

Clitoris: The highly sensitive organ located at the top of the vulva, where the labia minora meet. It plays a crucial role in sexual arousal and pleasure. See also *labia minora, vulva.*

Combination hormone therapy: A type of hormone therapy that includes both estrogen and progesterone. See also *estrogen, hormone therapy, progesterone.*

Corpus luteum: The sac that remains of the follicle in the ovary after ovulation takes place. The left-over corpus luteum, after the egg is released, produces progesterone after ovulation. The progesterone level stays elevated until a lack of fertilization triggers the next period, or it remains elevated if the egg is fertilized and implanted in the uterine wall. See also *follicle, ovaries, ovulation, progesterone.*

Deep vein thrombosis (DVT): Blood clots that form in the *veins* (blood vessels that bring blood toward the heart). A clot in one of these veins can be dangerous or even fatal if not detected and treated.

Dehydroepiandrosterone (DHEA): A hormone produced in the ovaries and adrenal glands of a woman, considered more *androgenic* (relating to male characteristic development) than estrogen or progesterone are. See also *androgens, estrogen, progesterone.*

Dual-energy X-ray absorptiometry (DEXA): A method of measuring the density of certain bones in the body — usually the lower spine, the hip, and the wrist — to screen for osteopenia and osteoporosis. See also *osteopenia, osteoporosis.*

Endocrine glands: Organs in the body that secrete hormones for use in the body by secreteing them into the bloodstream and affecting other (target) organs include the adrenal glands and the ovaries. See also *hormones, ovaries.*

Endometrium: The innermost lining of the uterus; the layer that sheds during menstruation. See also *menses, uterus.*

Estradiol: The active form of estrogen made in the ovaries prior to menopause. The most potent and abundant form of estrogen made in the body. See also *estrogen, menopause, ovaries.*

Estriol: A form of estrogen produced in the body mostly during pregnancy. In non-pregnant women, levels of estriol are usually low to undetectable. See also *estrogen.*

Estrogen: A hormone that, when present, promotes the development and maintenance of female characteristics of the body. Its irregularity and eventual absence plays a large part in perimenopause and menopause. See also *hormones.*

Estrogen receptor: A protein found on some cells that can bind to estrogen. When estrogen binds to a receptor, it triggers a series of cellular responses that can influence the activity of that cell. Two main types of estrogen receptors, ERα and ERβ, each have slightly different functions and tissue distributions. See also *estrogen.*

Estrone: A type of estrogen made by the ovaries, adrenal glands, and body fat prior to menopause. After menopause, the body's fatty tissues continue to make estrone. This is the only type of estrogen still naturally present after menopause. See also *estrogen.*

Fallopian tubes: A pair of hollow tube-like structures located between your ovaries and your uterus, through which an egg travels. See also *ovaries, uterus.*

Follicle: A small sac created in the ovary which grows and produces estrogen. At least one follicle per month releases an egg in someone who's ovulating regularly. After the follicle releases an egg, the remainder of the follicle is then called a *corpus luteum.* See also *corpus luteum, estrogen, ovary.*

Genitourinary Syndrome of Menopause (GSM): Formerly called *vulvovaginal atrophy* or *atrophic vaginitis,* this medical condition affects many women during perimenopause and menopause. GSM occurs due to a decrease in estrogen in the body, which affects the tissues of the vulva, vagina, and urinary system. These areas have many estrogen receptors, and when estrogen levels decline, these areas can get dry, irritated, and painful. See also *estrogen, estrogen receptors, vagina, vulva.*

High blood pressure: See *hypertension.*

High density lipoprotein (HDL): This type of cholesterol is considered good cholesterol because it helps carry fat from the body back to the liver for excretion. HDL plays a crucial role in the body's *lipid* (fat) metabolism. See also *cholesterol.*

Hormone therapy: Also called *menopausal hormone therapy.* Treatment with or use of hormones in perimenopause and menopause to relieve symptoms (typically hot flashes, night sweats, poor sleep, vaginal dryness, low energy, and mood swings) that occur in midlife and beyond. See also *hormones, menopause, perimenopause.*

Hormones: Chemicals produced in certain organs and glands in the body (called endocrine glands) that signal, activate, or moderate functions in other parts of the body. See also *endocrine glands.*

Hypertension: Commonly known as *high blood pressure.* A medical condition characterized by elevated blood pressure in the arteries. See also *blood pressure.*

Hysterectomy: Surgical removal of the uterus. See also *supracervical hysterectomy, total hysterectomy.*

Interstitial cystitis: A bladder condition that may be difficult to diagnose, but includes symptoms of pressure, mild discomfort, tenderness, and intense or chronic pain in the bladder and while urinating. You may need to urinate urgently and frequently, but a urinalysis shows no evidence of infection.

Introitus: The vaginal opening. See also *vagina*.

Labia: The lips of the vaginal opening, including the labia majora and the labia minora. The appearance of the labia can vary widely among individuals. See also *labia majora, labia minora*.

Labia majora: The larger outer folds of the labia, often covered with pubic hair, that protect the structures within. See also *labia*.

Labia minora: The two smaller, inner folds of the vaginal opening. They're thinner and more sensitive than the labia majora. See also *labia, labia majora*.

Libido: Your overall sexual drive or desire; the natural and psychological inclination toward engaging in sexual thoughts and behaviors. It can vary greatly among individuals, and a wide range of factors can influence it.

Low density lipoprotein (LDL): A type of lipoprotein in the bloodstream often referred to as bad cholesterol. It plays a role in transporting cholesterol from the liver to various cells and tissues in the body. Having too much LDL cholesterol in the bloodstream can lead to the buildup of cholesterol in the arteries. See also *cholesterol*.

Luteinizing hormone (LH): A hormone made in the pituitary gland of the brain. When released into the bloodstream, it has an effect on the ovaries, triggering ovulation. When you use a home ovulation predictor test, it checks for this LH surge to help you pinpoint when you're ovulating. See also *hormones, ovaries, ovulation*.

Menarche: The age of the onset of menstrual periods, usually around the age of 12, which signals the beginning of a woman's physical ability to reproduce.

Menopausal hormone therapy: See *hormone therapy*.

Menopause: The end of menstruation, fertility, and reproductive capability. Technically, no menstrual periods for 12 consecutive months. You can diagnose it only in retrospect, after 12 months with no periods have passed. The average age of menopause is 51. See also *menses*.

Menses: The periodic flow of blood from the uterus; also called a *period,* and generally occurring regularly and monthly during a woman's reproductive years. See also *uterus*.

Mixed incontinence: A form of urinary incontinence that combines elements of both stress incontinence and urge incontinence. See also *stress incontinence, urge incontinence, urinary incontinence*.

Oophorectomy: The surgical removal of one or both ovaries. This can be done as individual surgery or combined with a hysterectomy, with or without removal of the fallopian tubes. See also *bilateral salpingo-oophorectomy, fallopian tubes, hysterectomy*.

Osteoblast: A specialized bone cell responsible for bone formation and bone mineralization. These cells are crucial in the process of bone growth and development.

Osteoclast: These cells attach to the surface of bone tissue and secrete enzymes and acids that dissolve bone. This process breaks down and removes old and damaged bone tissue. Osteoclasts are essential for regulating calcium levels in the bloodstream.

Osteopenia: Loss of bone density not severe enough to be categorized as osteoporosis. If a person doesn't take action to maintain and strengthen the bone when diagnosed with osteopenia, over time, this condition evolves into osteoporosis. See also *osteoporosis.*

Osteoporosis: A medical condition characterized by the weakening of the bones, which then become fragile and more susceptible to fractures. Osteoporosis most commonly affects the hips, spine, and wrists. Often, this silent disease can progress without symptoms until a fracture occurs.

Ovaries: A pair of small, almond-shaped organs located in the female reproductive system responsible for releasing eggs during the menstrual cycle, travel into the fallopian tube and then the uterus, if fertilized. Ovaries also produce hormones — primarily estrogen and progesterone, but also testosterone. See also *estrogen, fallopian tubes, hormones, progesterone, testosterone.*

Ovulation: The process by which an egg is released from the follicle in the ovary. See also *follicle, ovaries.*

Pap smear: A procedure used to screen for abnormal changes in the cells of the cervix, primarily looking for pre-cancerous and cancerous changes to the cells. See also *cervix.*

Perimenopause: The time frame prior to menopause where hormone levels typically fluctuate, periods may become irregular, and other symptoms may occur, including emotional mood swings, poor sleep, heart palpitations, anxiety, irritability, vaginal dryness, hot flashes, and night sweats. It typically begins about four to six years prior to menopause but may last much longer. See also *hormones, menses, menopause.*

Perineum: The area of skin and tissue between the vaginal opening and the anus.

Polyp: A growth, usually non-cancerous, that protrudes from tissues. Polyps can form in the uterus and the cervix. See also *cervix, uterus.*

Postmenopause: The years after menopause begins, when the ovaries have stopped functioning; a time during which health conditions associated with long periods of low estrogen can cause major problems. See also *estrogen, menopause, ovaries.*

Premature menopause: Also called *premature ovarian failure.* Failure of the ovaries to function at an age that's much earlier than the average age of menopause. The ovaries stop their normal functions and stop developing follicles, releasing hormones, and ovulating. This condition can occur naturally or because of a medical condition, medications, surgery, or other medical treatments. Depending on the cause, it may or may not be reversible. See also *follicles, hormones, ovaries, ovulation.*

Premature ovarian failure: See *premature menopause.*

Progesterone: A female hormone produced by the ovaries after ovulation. It plays several important roles in the body, especially related to the menstrual cycle and pregnancy. It also contributes to bone health and mood stability. See also *hormones, menses, ovaries, ovulation.*

Progestin: A synthetic hormone that's similar in structure and function to progesterone. Medical professionals use progestins for many purposes, including contraception, menopausal hormone therapy, and infertility treatments. See also *hormones, hormone therapy, progesterone.*

Serotonin: A chemical messenger, called a *neurotransmitter,* which plays a crucial role in the functioning of the central nervous system. It influences mood regulation, sleep, appetite, and digestion, as well as behavior and emotions.

Stress incontinence: A form of urinary incontinence where you leak urine while doing activities such as laughing, jumping, coughing, or lifting something heavy. See also *urinary incontinence.*

Supracervical hysterectomy: Surgery to remove the body of the uterus, leaving the cervix in place. See also *cervix, hysterectomy, uterus.*

Surgical menopause: When menopause results from the surgical removal of the ovaries. See also *menopause, ovaries.*

Testosterone: A hormone primarily associated with male reproductive and sexual health and development. It's also present in females, but in smaller amounts. It belongs to the class of hormones called *androgens* and is thought to influence libido and sexual function, as well as muscle and bone health. See also *androgens, hormones, libido.*

Total hysterectomy: Surgical removal of the uterus and cervix. See also *cervix, hysterectomy uterus.*

Transdermal: A method by which you can deliver medications or drugs to your body through the skin. Patches, creams, and gels can deliver medication, especially hormones, by absorption through the skin so that they can go directly into the bloodstream. See also *hormones.*

Triglycerides: A type of fat found in the bloodstream that serves as a source of energy for various bodily functions. They're derived from the fats and oils that you consume in your diet, as well as excess sugar that your liver converts into triglycerides and stores in fat cells throughout your body. High levels of triglycerides can be a risk factor for heart disease.

Unopposed estrogen: A type of menopausal hormone therapy where a woman takes estrogen without also taking progesterone. With hormone therapy, if you take only estrogen, although it can relieve symptoms, it can also cause a buildup of tissue and endometrium inside the uterus. Progesterone can help eliminate or lessen this risk. Unopposed estrogen can result in the risk of a too-thick endometrial lining in the uterus, so doctors don't typically recommend an unopposed estrogen regimen for women who have a uterus (those who haven't had a hysterectomy). See also *endometrium, estrogen, hormone therapy, hysterectomy, progesterone, uterus.*

Urethra: The thin tube that runs from the bladder to the outside of your body, through which urine travels during urination.

Urge incontinence: A form of urinary incontinence where you experience an involuntary loss of urine, usually at random times or while on the way to the bathroom. See also *urinary incontinence*.

Urinary incontinence: The inability to maintain control over your bladder and urination.

Urinary tract infection (UTI): An infection that can affect the bladder (*cystitis*), the urethra (*urethritis*), or the kidneys (*pyelonephritis*). Bacteria makes its way into these organs and can cause symptoms such as a burning feeling when you urinate, needing to urinate frequently and urgently, noticing blood in the urine. If an infection reaches the kidneys, you can experience severe lower back pain and fever.

Vagina: A muscular tube leading from the cervix of the uterus to outside the body in women. See also *cervix, uterus*.

Vaginal atrophy: An outdated term for *Genitourinary Syndrome of Menopause*.

Vulva: The external part of the female genitals. It encompasses all the visible structures located on the outside of the body. See also *clitoris, introitus, labia, perineum, urethra*.

Vulvovaginal atrophy: An outdated term for *Genitourinary Syndrome of Menopause (GSM)*.

Appendix B

Perimenopause Resources

You can find a wealth of information on anything and everything you want to know about perimenopause and menopause, fitness, nutrition, hormones, medical screenings, and treatments. Here's a guide to some great resources — including books, articles, and online resources — that you may find helpful.

Books on Perimenopause and Related Issues

Each of the following books provide perspective and information that can help you navigate perimenopause and also ease your transition to menopause.

>> *The Blue Zones Secrets for Living Longer: Lessons From the Healthiest Places on Earth,* **by Dan Buettner (National Geographic):** An informative guide to the places on Earth where people live the longest. Includes the foods and behaviors that can help you live to be 100.

>> *Caring For Yourself While Caring for Your Aging Parents,* **by Claire Berman (Holt):** A practical guide to deal with all the issues you likely have to confront while caring for aging parents. This book addresses the wide range of emotions that can accompany caregiving, which can be even more stressful if you're going through perimenopause.

>> *The Menopause Manifesto: Own Your Own Health With Facts and Feminism,* **by Dr Jen Gunter (Citadel):** This book will bring you empowerment through knowledge by countering many of the stubborn myths and misunderstandings about menopause with hard facts and science.

>> *Next Level: Your Guide to Kicking Ass, Feeling Great and Crushing Goals Through Menopause and Beyond,* **by Stacy Sims and Selene Yeager (Rodale Books):** A comprehensive guide to peak performance for active women approaching or experiencing menopause.

>> *Track the Perimenopause: Record Your Cycle, Symptoms, Sleep and Mood,* **by A.F. White (Medjournal Lifeseries):** A year-long symptom tracker that helps you easily record your cycle, symptoms, sleep, and moods, designed specifically for perimenopause. Use the information that you record to decide how to best care for yourself.

>> *What Fresh Hell Is This? Perimenopause, Menopause, Other Indignities and You,* **by Heather Corinna (Hatchette Go):** An informative, blisteringly funny, cranky guide to perimenopause and menopause by an award-winning sex and health educator.

>> *You've Got to Be Kidding Me! Perimenopause Symptoms, Stages and Strategies,* **by Jen Sweeney (BookBaby):** A comprehensive, concise, and easy-to-read guide that combines personal anecdotes with research to demystify this significant stage in women's lives.

Websites, Articles, and Online Resources

The following list of articles, websites, and other online resources can help you find information you need about perimenopause and related mental and physical health support.

>> **American Psychological Association (APA):** You can find a wealth of psychological research offering insights on how women can experience the perimenopausal transition with greater comfort and insight. On the APA website (www.apa.org), simply enter "menopause" into the search text box to access your options.

>> **The Canadian Menopause Society:** A non-profit organization consisting of medical professionals interested in perimenopausal and menopausal health (www.sigmamenopause.com).

>> **Centers for Disease Control and Prevention (CDC):** You can find basic information about reproductive cancers — diagnosis, treatment, prognosis — by searching for "gynecological cancer" on the main website (www.cdc.gov).

>> **The Endocrine Society:** Endocrinologists specialize in the treatment of metabolic disorders, diabetes, and menopause. On the main page of the Endocrine Society (`www.endocrine.org`), search for "menopause" to access many great resources related to menopause.

>> **Everyday Health:** On the main website (`www.everydayhealth.com`), enter the search term "perimenopause" to find all kinds of articles and information about this stage in your life.

>> **"Exercising with osteoporosis," by the Mayo Clinic (`www.mayoclinic.org`):** This article offers information on how certain types of exercise can strengthen muscles and bones while other types can improve balance, which can help prevent falls.

>> **Gennev:** The largest virtual menopause clinic in the United States (`www.gennev.com`). You can access information about evidence-based treatments from board-certified OB/GYNs and dietitians in relation to perimenopause and menopause by clicking the Learn link at the top of the main page. And click the For Patients link to figure out whether you can receive medical treatment for your symptoms, all from the comfort of home.

>> **"How to Sleep Better During Perimenopause," by Christina Ianzito:** This article appears on the AARP website (`www.aarp.org`). From the main page, click the search icon and enter "sleep during perimenopause" in the search text box. This article should appear near the top of the results, offering some better ways to calm restless nights.

>> **The Menopause Society:** Formerly the North American Menopause Society, this nonprofit organization serves as the definitive resource for healthcare professionals and the public for accurate information on menopause and healthy aging. Its site (`www.menopause.org`) also has a feature where you can find a menopause specialist near you. From the main site, select For Women ⇨ Find a Menopause Practitioner.

>> **The Midst:** An online information source and community for health and wellness over 40 (`http://themidst.substack.com`).

>> **The National Institute on Aging:** On the main website (`www.nia.nih.gov`), enter "menopause" in the search text box to access information that can help you understand menopause and the menopausal transition.

>> **Our Bodies Ourselves:** This evidence-based feminist resource (`www.ourbodiesourselves.org`) is aimed at demystifying perimenopause and destigmatizing menopause.

>> **"Perimenopause Explained," by Carrie St. Michel:** An interview with several OB/GYNs about various symptoms and treatments for perimenopause available from the Cedars-Sinai website (`www.cedars-sinai.org`); search for "perimenopause explained" on the main page and then select the Articles tab on the results page to access a link to this article.

Alternatives to Hormones

This book talks about several alternatives to hormone treatments, which I list in the following sections. Always speak to your doctor before taking anything to treat perimenopause symptoms.

For hot flashes

The following can be helpful when dealing with hot flashes.

>> **Equelle (www.equelle.com):** A supplement containing S-equol, which shares a similar molecular structure to estrogen; take two tablets per day.

>> **Estrovera (www.metagenics.com/estrovera):** A plant-based formula called ERr 731, made from the root of a rhubarb plant; take one tablet per day.

>> **Relizen (www.hellobonafide.com/relizen):** A plant-based formula including Swedish flower pollen; take two tablets per day, with or without food.

>> **Tempo (www.pronovacorp.com):** From the Pronova main page, select the Menopause option at the top of the screen, then choose Tempo Hot Flashes. This supplement uses *genistein* (the primary *isoflavone,* or plant-based compound that can mimic estrogen, found in soy); take one tablet per day.

For vaginal dryness

If you are experiencing the discomfort of vaginal dryness, you may find relief with the following products.

>> **Hyalogyn (www.hyalogyn.com):** A personal vaginal moisturizer to increase the comfort of sexual activity. It contains hyaluronic acid. Comes in gel and suppositories.

>> **K-Y Liquibeads (www.k-y.com):** From the main page, click the search icon and enter "liquibeads" for the product to appear as a result. It comes in an ovule that dissolves within minutes and provides a personal lubricant with moisture for up to 48 hours.

>> **Revaree (www.hellobonafide.com/revaree):** A vaginal insert to increase moisture for vaginal comfort with intimacy. Made with hyaluronic acid, which improves the tissue's ability to retain water.

>> **Via (www.solvwellness.com):** Click the Via link at the top of the main page to access information about this cream moisturizer specifically designed to be absorbed by the vaginal and vulvar tissues. It contains hyaluronic acid, CoQ10, and vitamins E and C.

Index

brain fog, 119–128
  benefits of exercise, 204
  evaluating causes of, 14
  forgetfulness, 122
  improving cognitive function, 123–125
  medications affecting, 126–127
  memory boost, 128
  mood shifts, 122
  multitasking, 121
  overview, 35
  regulating body temperature, 121–122
  sleep cycle, 122
  as symptom of perimenopause, 10
BRCA 1 and 2 (breast cancer susceptibility gene), 42–43
breakthrough bleeding, 80
breast cancer, 42–43, 239, 267–268
breastfeeding, 76
bremelanotide, 110
Brisdelle (paroxetine), 93, 126, 141
bruising, 24
building bones, 224–225
bulimia, 58
bupropion (Wellbutrin), 141

C

calcium, 22, 197–198, 230–232
Calm website, 139
calmness, 149–150
calorie deficit, 200
cancer, 238–240
  breast cancer, 239
  cervical cancer, 240
  colorectal cancer, 238–239
  detecting precancerous cells, 266–267
cancerous cells, 70
carbamazepine (Tegretol), 159
carbohydrates, 190–191
Catapres (clonidine), 92
Caucasian women, 227
CBC (complete blood count), 240–241
CBT (cognitive behavioral therapy), 131, 138
central sleep apnea (CSA), 161
cervical cancer, 240

cervix
  abnormal cells on, 70
  overview, 68
cheat sheet for book, 4
chemotherapy, 46–47, 56
chest fly, 215
childbirth, 176
chin hair, 24–25
Chinese women, 8–9
cholesterol, 21, 108, 238
clarity, 86
climate control, 153
clonidine (Catapres), 92
codeine, 127
cognitive behavioral therapy (CBT), 131, 138
cognitive function, 35, 123–125
collagen, 24
cologuard test, 239
colonoscopy, 239
colorectal cancer, 238–239
colposuspension, 183
combination pills, 79–81, 88
communication, 258
  about low libido, 100–101
  establishing open channels of, 153
  maintaining healthy boundaries, 146
  with partner about perimenopause symptoms, 16–17
complete blood count (CBC), 240–241
complex atypical hyperplasia, 267
complex carbohydrates, 190–191
complex sleep apnea (treatment-emergent sleep apnea), 161
concentration, 10, 14
continuous dosing, 81
continuous positive airway pressure (CPAP) device, 160
conventional dosing, 80
cooling lubricants, 104
coronary artery disease, 237–238
corpus luteum cyst, 71
cortisol, 131
counseling, 137–138
couples therapy, 109, 114, 115
CPAP (continuous positive airway pressure) device, 160
cream, estrogen, 102
crow's feet, 24

fruits, 191

FSH. *See* follicle-stimulating hormone (FSH)

fundus, 68

G

GABA (gamma-amino-butyric acid), 157, 163

gabapentin, 92

gabapentin enacarbil (Horizant), 159

generalized vulvodynia, 112

genetic mutation, 42–43

genistein, 91

genital discomfort

  evaluating causes of, 14

  libido and, 104–105

  as symptom of perimenopause, 10

genitourinary syndrome of menopause (GSM), 26, 101–102

German measles, 236

ginseng, 91

glucose, 40, 120

growth, bones, 224–225

H

habits, 56–60

  alcohol intake, 57–58

  exercise, 59–60, 205

  extreme weight fluctuation, 58

  healthy eating, 188–190

    identifying social and emotional eating, 190

    perimenopausal transition diet, 189

  medical conditions, 57

  medications, 56–57

  smoking, 56

  surgeries, 58–59

hair distribution, 23–25

HDL (high-density lipoprotein), 194, 238

Headspace website, 139

health screenings. *See* screening tests

healthcare providers. *See* medical practitioners

heart attacks, 21

heart center, 151

heart health

  benefits of exercise, 206

  libido and, 106, 108

  overview, 21

  severe hot flashes and, 33

heart palpitations

  evaluating causes of, 12–13

  as symptom of perimenopause, 9

heart rate, 209–211

heart rate monitor, 210–211

heavier periods, 66

heavy sudden bleeding, 68

herbs, 110

herpes genitals, 105

high blood pressure, 237

high-density lipoprotein (HDL), 194, 238

high-intensity workouts, 210

hippocampus, 125

Hispanic women, 8–9

histamine blockers, 108

Horizant (gabapentin enacarbil), 159

hormonal IUDs (progesterone releasing IUDs), 82, 89

hormone replacement therapy (HRT), 84

hormone therapy

  alternatives to, 89–93

    prescription medications, 91–93

    supplements, 90–91

  for anxiety, 131

  brain fog and, 124

  correcting bleeding patterns, 72

  cyclic estrogen and progesterone, 87–88

  cyclic progesterone, 87

  daily progesterone, 87

  hot flashes and, 264

  menopausal hormone therapy, 88–89

  progesterone, 85–86

  risk of cancer and, 43

  surgical menopause, 45–46

hormone-blocking drugs, 228

hormones, 73–93

  affecting sleep, 156–161, 164–165

    estrogen, 165

    hot flashes, 157

    insomnia, 158

    progesterone, 164–165

    restless leg syndrome, 158–159

    sleep apnea, 159–161

O

obesity, 17, 58, 160, 236
obstructive sleep apnea (OSA), 160–161
oil-based lubricants, 104
omega-3 fatty acids, 194
omega-6 fatty acids, 194
online forums, 253
online references, 280–281
  cheat sheet for book, 4
  mindfulness, 139
  therapists, 138
oophorectomy, 59
opioids, 108
organ function tests, 237–238
  blood pressure, 237
  lipid panel, 237–238
orthosomnia, 167
OSA (obstructive sleep apnea), 160–161
osteoblasts, 224
osteoclasts, 224
osteopenia, 196, 224
osteoporosis, 22, 196–197, 205, 224
OTC (over-the-counter) sleep aids, 169–170
ovarian cancer, 42–43
ovarian cysts, 70, 105
ovaries
  hysterectomy, 44
  overview, 69
  polycystic ovarian syndrome, 38–40
    adrenal PCOS, 40
    inflammatory PCOS, 40
    insulin-resistant PCOS, 39–40
    post-pill PCOS, 40
  premature ovarian failure, 41–42
  progesterone produced in, 75
  removal of, 45
overactive bladder (urge incontinence), 23, 177
overflow incontinence, 179
over-the-counter (OTC) sleep aids, 169–170
ovulation, 28
  hormone stability during, 30
  irregular, 71
  overview, 27
oxybutynin (Oxytrol), 126, 184
oxycodone, 127

P

pain medications, 127
Pamelor (nortriptyline), 126–127
pancreas, 40
Pap smears, 240
parathyroid glands, 230
paroxetine, 93, 126, 141
patch, birth control, 81–82
Patient Health Questionnaire-9 (PHQ-9), 237
PCOS. *See* polycystic ovarian syndrome (PCOS)
pelvic floor conditions, 105
pelvic floor physical therapy, 180
pelvic inflammatory disease (PID), 76
pelvic muscles, 180–182
percutaneous tibial nerve stimulation (PTNS), 185
perforations, 42
perimenopausal rage, 135
perimenopause, 7–18
  calling in professionals, 17–18
  causes of bleeding patterns during, 68–72
    anatomical changes, 69–70
    combination of factors, 72
    hormonal changes, 72
    irregular ovulation, 71
  misinformation about, 251–256
  myths about, 245–250
    asking for help, 249
    bladder issues, 248
    checking hormone levels, 250
    irregular vaginal bleeding, 247
    menopausal symptoms in perimenopause, 247
    pregnancy, 250
    sexual activity, 246
    using hormones when in menopause, 246
    waiting out symptoms, 249
    weight gain, 248
  overview, 7
  physical changes in, 17
  recognizing difference between other conditions and, 11–17
    evaluating causes of symptoms, 11–15
    talking about symptoms, 15–17
  symptoms of, 9–10
  women of color and, 7–8
pertussis, 236

symptoms
- common, 9–10
- myths about, 249
- recognizing difference between other conditions and perimenopause, 11–17
  - evaluating causes of symptoms, 11–15
  - talking about symptoms, 15–17
- treating with hormones, 84–89
  - hormone therapies, 86–88
  - menopausal hormone therapy, 88–89
  - progesterone, 85–86

systolic pressure, 237

T

tablets, estrogen, 103
tai chi, 208
tampons, incontinence, 182
target heart rate, 211
Tegretol (carbamazepine), 159
temazepam (Restoril), 127
temperature control, 153
Tempo, 91
tennis, 206
testosterone, 32, 266
- for hypoactive sexual desire disorder, 110–111
- with menopause hormone therapy, 88

tetanus, 236
thyroid function
- brain fog caused by, 35
- irregular cycles due to, 76
- libido and, 106
- screening tests for, 240

time zones, 76
tolterodine (Detrol), 126, 184
topiramate (Topamax), 93
torsion, 45
Toviaz (fesoterodine), 184
tracking sleep apps, 166
tracking technology, 167
training bladder, 186
tramadol, 127
trans fats, 193–194
transdermal estrogen, 45, 88
travel, 76

treatment-emergent sleep apnea (complex sleep apnea), 161
triceps kickback, 217–218
triglycerides, 238
tryptophan, 164
tubal ligation, 83
Type 1 diabetes, 57
Type 2 diabetes, 40, 57, 236

U

unprovoked vulvodynia, 113
unsaturated fats, 194–195
ureters, 175
urethra, 10, 22, 175
urge incontinence (overactive bladder), 23, 177
urinary retention, 185
urinary tract, 174–175. See also bladder issues
urinary tract infections (UTIs), 23, 178
urodynamics, 184–185
uterine lining
- doctor checking, 39
- endometrial ablation, 41–42
- fibroids in, 53–54
- during menstrual cycle, 74

uterus, 68–69

V

vaccinations, 236
vagina
- changes in, 25–26
- evaluating causes of discomfort, 14
- overview, 69
- symptom of perimenopause and, 10

vaginal atrophy, 26
vaginal estrogen products, 102–103
vaginal pain conditions, 112–115
- dryness, 186, 282
- libido and, 104–105
- vaginismus, 114–115
- vulvodynia, 112–114
  - causes of, 113–114
  - treating, 114

vaginal pessary, 182–183

About the Author

Dr. Rebecca Levy-Gantt grew up in Brooklyn, New York, where she enjoyed playing softball and was a voracious reader. She earned a Bachelor's Degree in Health Sciences before moving to Boston to attend Boston University, studying physical therapy and graduating with a Master's Degree. While in graduate school, she reconsidered her life plan, quietly deciding to apply for medical school. She moved back to New York, and while working as a physical therapist, she returned to night school to prepare for the MCAT, the medical school admission test.

She continued to be interested in rehabilitation science and was planning to focus on the specialty of Physical Medicine and Rehabilitation. She believed in the philosophy of looking at the "whole person" and applied to osteopathic medical schools, where that seemed to be the prevailing philosophy.

Over the first few years of studying medicine, life circumstances changed, and she had two children — a boy and a girl — while in school. These life events delayed her studies a bit, but also affected her choice of specialty. Dr. Levy-Gantt published a book about her experiences in medical school and beyond, called *Womb With A View*, in 2020 (Wordrunner Press). By the time she graduated from medical school, Dr. Levy-Gantt was sure that obstetrics and gynecology was her calling.

Levy-Gantt has now been practicing for 30 years, first in New York, then in California. She has a wonderful husband, Bill, who has supported her career and her writing, and they have a son, the third child for each of them. She loves to run, travel, write — and most of all, provide comprehensive care to women in her medical practice.

Dedication

To Bill: A momentary chance encounter; a lifetime of devotion, passion, family fun, and entertainment.

Acknowledgements

Special thanks to my tribe: my women friends whom I have counted on to read my words, discuss ideas, contribute knowledge, support my work, and most of all, talk me down from the ledge: Patty DeRosa, Karen Hillman, Lori Lieberman, Laura Paoletti, Lili Garcia, Ditza Katz, Ross Tabisel, and Danielle Bezalel (my daughter *and* my friend).

And thank you to the thousands of patients I've cared for over the last 30 years, for helping me figure out the right way to care for you all and having a great time in the process.

Thank you to my team at Wiley, including my editors, copy editor, and proofreader, and everyone who has given me this great opportunity, guiding me and helping me on the journey to create this book.

Publisher's Acknowledgments

Acquisitions Editor: Jennifer Yee

Project Manager: Tracy Brown

Copy Editor: Laura Miller

Technical Editor: Shelley Dolitsky

Senior Managing Editor: Kristie Pyles

Proofreader: Susan Hobbs

Production Editor: Saikarthick Kumarasamy

Cover Image: © Carlos Barquero/Getty Images

Take dummies with you everywhere you go!

Whether you are excited about e-books, want more from the web, must have your mobile apps, or are swept up in social media, dummies makes everything easier.

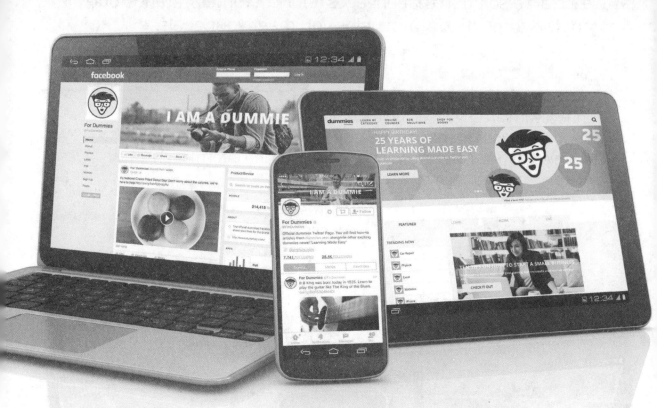

Find us online!

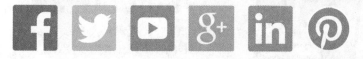

dummies.com

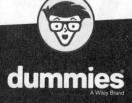

Leverage the power

Dummies is the global leader in the reference category and one of the most trusted and highly regarded brands in the world. No longer just focused on books, customers now have access to the dummies content they need in the format they want. Together we'll craft a solution that engages your customers, stands out from the competition, and helps you meet your goals.

Advertising & Sponsorships

Connect with an engaged audience on a powerful multimedia site, and position your message alongside expert how-to content. Dummies.com is a one-stop shop for free, online information and know-how curated by a team of experts.

- Targeted ads
- Video
- Email Marketing
- Microsites
- Sweepstakes sponsorship

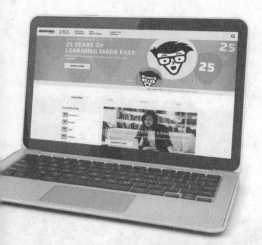

20 MILLION PAGE VIEWS EVERY SINGLE MONTH

15 MILLION UNIQUE VISITORS PER MONTH

43% OF ALL VISITORS ACCESS THE SITE VIA THEIR MOBILE DEVICES

700,000 NEWSLETTER SUBSCRIPTIONS

TO THE INBOXES OF

300,000 UNIQUE INDIVIDUALS EVERY WEEK

# of dummies

Custom Publishing

Reach a global audience in any language by creating a solution that will differentiate you from competitors, amplify your message, and encourage customers to make a buying decision.

- Apps
- Books
- eBooks
- Video
- Audio
- Webinars

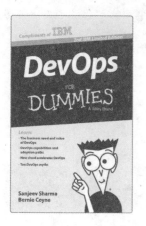
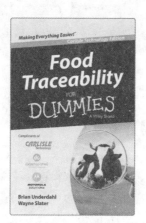
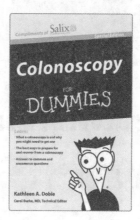
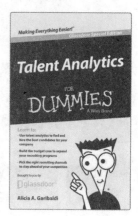

Brand Licensing & Content

Leverage the strength of the world's most popular reference brand to reach new audiences and channels of distribution.

For more information, visit **dummies.com/biz**

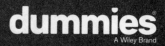

PERSONAL ENRICHMENT

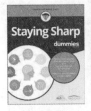
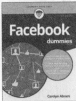
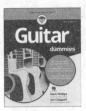
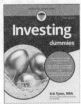
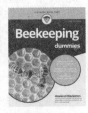
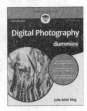

9781119187790	9781119179030	9781119293354	9781119293347	9781119310068	9781119235606
USA $26.00	USA $21.99	USA $24.99	USA $22.99	USA $22.99	USA $24.99
CAN $31.99	CAN $25.99	CAN $29.99	CAN $27.99	CAN $27.99	CAN $29.99
UK £19.99	UK £16.99	UK £17.99	UK £16.99	UK £16.99	UK £17.99

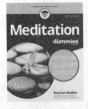
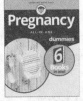
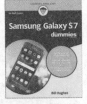
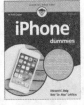
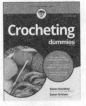
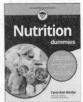

9781119251163	9781119235491	9781119279952	9781119283133	9781119287117	9781119130246
USA $24.99	USA $26.99	USA $24.99	USA $24.99	USA $24.99	USA $22.99
CAN $29.99	CAN $31.99	CAN $29.99	CAN $29.99	CAN $29.99	CAN $27.99
UK £17.99	UK £19.99	UK £17.99	UK £17.99	UK £16.99	UK £16.99

PROFESSIONAL DEVELOPMENT

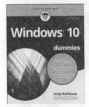

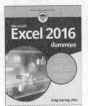
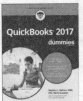
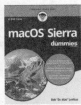
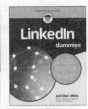

9781119311041	9781119255796	9781119293439	9781119281467	9781119280651	9781119251132	9781119310563
USA $24.99	USA $39.99	USA $26.99	USA $26.99	USA $29.99	USA $24.99	USA $34.00
CAN $29.99	CAN $47.99	CAN $31.99	CAN $31.99	CAN $35.99	CAN $29.99	CAN $41.99
UK £17.99	UK £27.99	UK £19.99	UK £19.99	UK £21.99	UK £17.99	UK £24.99

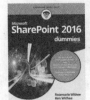
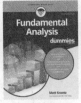

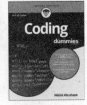

9781119181705	9781119263593	9781119257769	9781119293477	9781119265313	9781119239314	9781119293323
USA $29.99	USA $26.99	USA $29.99	USA $26.99	USA $24.99	USA $29.99	USA $29.99
CAN $35.99	CAN $31.99	CAN $35.99	CAN $31.99	CAN $29.99	CAN $35.99	CAN $35.99
UK £21.99	UK £19.99	UK £21.99	UK £19.99	UK £17.99	UK £21.99	UK £21.99

dummies.com

dummies®
A Wiley Brand